Standing The Watch

Standing The Watch

Memories of a home death

Rebecca Brown

Writer's Showcase
San Jose New York Lincoln Shanghai

Standing The Watch
Memories of a home death

All Rights Reserved © 2002 by Rebecca Brown

No part of this book may be reproduced or transmitted in any form or by any means, graphic, electronic, or mechanical, including photocopying, recording, taping, or by any information storage retrieval system, without the permission in writing from the publisher.

Writer's Showcase
an imprint of iUniverse, Inc.

For information address:
iUniverse, Inc.
5220 S. 16th St., Suite 200
Lincoln, NE 68512
www.iuniverse.com

Quotations from *The Power of Myth* by Joseph Campbell and Bill Moyers reprinted by permission from Doubleday.
Quotation from *When the Drummers Were Women* by Layne Redmond reprinted by permission of Three Rivers Press and the author.

Cover photographs: Rebecca Brown
Illustrations:
Townsend's Chipmunk Image Copyright 2002 by Wanda Krick, Artist.
Steller's Blue Jay Image, Copyright 2002 Wild Birds Unlimited, Inc., Rebecca Moore Higgins, Artist.

Read this book before your parents die!

ISBN: 0-595-22750-3

Printed in the United States of America

Percival Vivian Burnett
1896-1957
who took this child under his wing
Lincoln Brown
1910-1999
who gave this woman a father again
Michael John Barbee
1953-2001
who was a brother to this sister
Good men and fathers, too!

Percival Vivian Burnett took me in as a yearling during WWII, and adopted me after VE Day. He gave me a new name, a home, a family, and the love of reading and writing. He was proud to be the first Jew ever accepted as a Fellow of the Royal Institute of British Architects.
Lincoln Brown came into my life when I was fifty and gave me a father again. He often thanked me for my care, and would bring me the first ripe tomatoes and raspberries. It was a joy to hear him learn to say "I love you."
Michael John Barbee brought into our lives sunshine and eagles, tie-dyed shirts and crystals, wood stoves and water fountains and, when we were building Poppa's cabin, his willing hands and strength. He was a Spirit Brother to my husband, and a Brother to my Heart.

Contents

Foreword ....*ix*

Thank you to... ....*xiii*

Beginnings: Promise me! *3*

The Us of Us: Honoring our vows *17*

Day 1: Our paths into The Valley *29*

Day 3: Daddy's home! *47*

Day 5: Good morning, Sweetheart! *53*

Day 6: The Certificate of Impending Death *69*

Our Gift: They don't make house calls *81*

Day 7: Hear, O Lord, when I cry. *91*

Day 8: With all my fingers and toes *101*

Day 9: A closer walk with Poppa *109*

Day 10: Uphill and into the wind *115*

Day 11: A nickel's worth of five dollar bills *125*

Day 12: Famous last words *131*

Day 13: He restoreth my soul 139

Lessons: Dying to learn 149

How then will we die?: Another sunrise 165

Connections: And life goes on 173

Another gift from the Cosmos 181

The Days of Lincoln Brown: 1910-1999 189

A passel of comforting books 191

About the Author 203

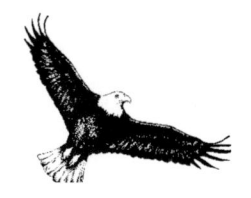

Foreword

by Lynn Lott, M.A., M.F.T.

I remember a time when my mother replied to a comment I made about how sad I would be to lose her saying, "Lynn, no one is put on this earth to live forever." As a person who has lived most of my life in as much denial as I can muster about death, Rebecca Brown's book *Standing the Watch: Memories of a home death*, was just what I needed to wake me up and reeducate me about dying and death.

Before reading this book, I never believed that giving a loved-one a home death could be a gift to both the dying and the living. Oh sure, I'd heard countless people tell me how glad they were to be with a loved-one as they passed from this world, how special the experience was, and how they underwent their own spiritual high. Did I believe them? No way! But now, after reading Rebecca's book, I'm wondering.

I have experienced several home births, never questioning the rightness of being present when someone draws their first breath, yet I have lived in fear of being present when someone draws their last. Is this because I think they aren't worth it? No. Is it because I think dying is best done in a hospital? No. It's simply because it's unknown to me and therefore, I'm scared.

Standing The Watch has helped me feel less fearful, as I could be an invisible fly on the wall as Rebecca and David ministered to her dying father-in-law. After accompanying them on their journey, I can believe Rebecca when she says, "While a home death can be frightening, time-consuming, worrying, stressful, unpleasant and tedious, it is also a fertile ground for courage, discipline, stamina, spirituality, compassion, loyalty, humor and love."

With a combination of stories, logs, e-mails, childhood memories and essays of microscopic honesty, Rebecca takes us on the journey of her father-in-law, Lincoln Brown's last days. As you read you'll feel like you are chatting with Rebecca over a cup of tea. Her style is warm, loving, informative and awe-inspiring. It is no surprise that she received a lot of encouragement from her friends to write this book. By making the time in her life to put down this story of dying and death, she helps all of us learn to accept that death is as natural a part of life as birth.

Why would we want to learn more about death? As a writer of parenting and other self-help books, I know there is no shortage of books teaching us how to welcome, celebrate and live life. But we still hide from death or hope others will take care of it for us. As one of Rebecca's friends said, "I am always surprised how few people realize the sacredness of death, what an honor it is to be present...By attending to death with the same seriousness as birth, we learn how to die."

Whether you intend to care for a loved-one as they die and are looking for comfort, wisdom and help, or whether you doubt that you will ever be at the bedside of a dying person, there is much to gain from Rebecca Brown's book. Surely, you will be swept away by the love that fills the pages. Absolutely, you will be amazed at the courage and tenacity of David and Rebecca as they help Lincoln exit this world. And certainly, you will be comforted by the stories of other deaths and other times as Rebecca shares from her past. I am guessing you will find yourself thinking, "I wish I could be like that." Or, "I could never be like that." Or, "Lincoln Brown was one lucky man." I promise that your feelings will be stirred and you will be lovingly nurtured out of your denial of death.

I highly recommend you spend an evening or two with this book, in front of the fire if you have one. The time you spend will be enriching both in the present while you are captivated by Rebecca Brown's story, and in the future, when you are experiencing a death of a loved-one, or perhaps, even your own. Since we aren't put on this earth to live forever, we can face death with more courage, honesty and acceptance after reading *Standing The Watch: Memories of a home death*.

I personally would like to thank Rebecca for writing her own story, in addition to all the writing she does about our books. She has many gifts, especially this ability to take on the unspoken and tell it like it is.

Lynn Lott is a sought-after therapist, motivational speaker, frequent TV talk show guest, and prolific writer. She has written many books, five manuals for teachers and parent educators, and has contributed articles to numerous magazines, newspapers, and online publications. Her most notable works include: *Chores Without Wars*, *Positive Discipline A-Z*, and *Do-It-Yourself Therapy*.

Thank you to...

David H., for being a loving husband, nag, mentor, intrepid computer and cyberspace explorer, creator of my own website, and urging me to write, write, write.

Ben and Rayna Burnett, loving son and daughter-in-law, for their vital support during the writing of this book.

Alice Keene-Kadel, my lifelong friend, who supported my adventures, both in spirit and finances.

My Reading Group for their encouragement: Lynn Lott, Carolyn Stearns, C. J. Macgenn and C. Lynwood Sawyer.

My cyberspace friends for being there when I needed them: Ruth Raven, May Tracer, Jane Hall, Deborah Daubner-Michel, Faina, Artie Carter, and Donna Klopfer.

Del and Nancy Alsop who heard a brother's plea.

Wanda Krick for her artwork, supplies of organic eggs and surprise meals, and eager ear for my adventures.

Pam Carlson, R.N., bearer of hands-on validation.

David and I could not have made it without the help of these folks: Char at the DSHS/CA in Forks; ParaTransit of Western Washington; Clallam Home Health in Port Angeles; Jim's Pharmacy in Port Angeles and Chinook Pharmacy in Forks.

To my Sponsors, without whom this book would not have made it to print: Ben and Rayna Burnett; Nancy and Delbert Alsop; Victor and Cookie Cohen; Carolyn Stearns; Jeremy and Adrie Burnett; Carolyn Starr; Deborah and William Daubner-Michel; Jane Hall, and Dr. Alma Bond.

Standing The Watch

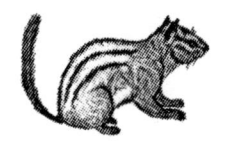

Beginnings

Promise me!

"We all need to tell our story and...to understand...to cope with death...we all need help in our passages from birth to life and then to death. We need for life to signify, to touch the eternal, to understand the mysterious, to find out who we are."
Bill Moyers, *The Power of Myth*

Today, more often than not, we meet death as we greet birth, as names on the rosters of professional shift-changing strangers in distant institutions. Choosing to die at home seems to be an embarrassment, an imposition, which I discovered when no one at the clinic or hospital wanted to talk with us about our choice.

Anytime of the day or night on television, there are ads showing nice, elderly folks making arrangements so as not to burden their children with their final months, weeks, days and hours here on Earth. Who then will learn about dying?

In the course of Standing The Watch for my husband's father's dying, I was to learn the lessons of frustration and endurance, dread and bewilderment, humor and compassion. I also felt I was being given an opportunity to heal a lifelong wound. My husband and I both knew we were in the presence of the sacred, the prosaic and the eternal.

Standing The Watch is about honoring a vow a son made to his father. That vow stretched us way beyond our comfort levels until we forgot to eat, and were catching naps during the dissolved nights and days. In keeping that vow, we uncovered insights into our weaknesses and our strengths, and our ideas about responsibility. We stepped into deep moments of affection and contentment; we stumbled into lighter ones of relief, grace and humor. We pulled together in the traces of our marriage, holding each other's hand like the little girl and little boy we were, walking into the inevitable shadows of our mortality to catch glimpses of the Mystery of Spirit.

Blessed are the children who care for their parents, for they will be loved by their ancestors and their descendants. What else is there than to be loved?

*   *   *   *   *

On a cool and wet June day in 1957, when I was fourteen years old, the father of my childhood took his children to the Commonwealth Games at the White City Arena in London, after which we all came down with summer colds. All recovered except Father.

After my end-of-summer birthday, I returned to my day school, the only child still at home. By October, Mother murmured, in our hushed home, that Father would not be recovering. A nurse was hired to attend him, and I helped Mother move into her boudoir-cum-sewing room to make way for the medical contraptions.

Each Friday evening, as the grandfather clock chimed the hour, Mother would unlock the front door and retreat to the dining room and her knitting. I would settle on a step in the curve of the stairway behind the ornate balustrade, and watch as a *minyon* of Homburg-hatted, black-coated men quietly entered our home and walked into the sitting room directly beneath my parents' bedroom. After the door closed, a silence lay heavily in our home, until I would hear the first deep voice raised in prayer. For an hour, our home was filled with those prayers. The darkened niche in which I crouched, seemed to lighten and often, as those deep voices rose and fell, I'd doze, imagining I was once again in my Daddy's lap, listening to him speak.

In time, the chanting would fade away, and the men would file out into the hallway, hats and coats already on, and quietly leave our house. Then Mother would come out of her retreat and lock up after them. I would creep back up to my room. My mother and I never spoke about those evening prayers.

I was only once permitted to see Daddy during those months. At my begging, Mother had pushed me, alone, into their room where the nurse silently sat in a dimly lit corner. The gas fire had made the air stifling. Father lay shrunken and sunken in their vast bed.

What was I supposed to do? Might I sit on the bed and talk to him? Tell him about my day, as I had done, at his request, for so many years? Could he hear me? Was he in pain? Who to ask? When I looked over at the nurse, she shook her head, and remained silent. For fear of doing something wrong, I simply stood, touching my father's hand, glancing up at his face, almost hidden by the pillows and bedclothes, listening to his shallow breathing. All I could do was remember him in my life, and wonder about this thing called Death.

By midwinter, the end was near. My mother and I had half-heartedly put up the holiday decorations. No one brought home a tree, because that had been our Daddy's pride and joy. Then my mother had covered everything, even the mirrors, with swatches of black cloth. Soon, all my brothers had come home, my oldest with his new wife, my middle one in his National Service uniform, and my youngest from boarding school. No one felt like going through the rituals that our family had enjoyed all my childhood. We exchanged gifts on Christmas morning with somber thanks, and the dinner that evening, was silently eaten. The traditional crackers, bright holiday toys which we enjoyed popping at meal's end, were left on the table.

On Boxing Day morning, my youngest brother's birthday, Mother woke me with the news that Daddy had died in the night and all was over. Before lunch time, I had been told I was too young for what was to come, and to pack my suitcase because Jo Hyde-Smith, a longtime family friend, would be collecting me to spend the rest of the holidays in Blackheath, on the other side of London.

Jo had lived next door to us for years, and had often given me a safe haven, had been my other mother, when tensions torqued at home. When her husband, Sam, suddenly died, she had moved away. At least once a year, I had visited her, and I noticed how no one spoke of Sam.

Each lonely day in her home that winter, as I helped her with her children, I wondered about death, and why I had been exiled from my family. When I returned home, all traces of my Daddy had gone, and all photographs of him had vanished. My parents' bedroom had been put back in place. I quickly learnt that any mention of Daddy was taboo, and no one then ever told me where he had been buried.

It was more than three decades later, with my own children full grown, that a firm of solicitors from England found me in America to tell me that my mother had died. On my return to the land of my childhood, I visited with my brothers' families. Eventually I learnt what had happened to my parents' remains: my mother's ashes had been strewn over the Sussex seashore she had so loved, and my father had been interred in the Golders Green Cemetery. One cold and sunny January day, I set out to find my father's grave. With my grown-up daughter, I paid my long overdue respects, and placed upon his gravestone three pebbles I had brought from the beaches beside my Northwest home, one for each of his grandchildren and one from his grateful daughter.

Then I returned to my full life in America where the Cosmos had brought David and me together through our Paths to the Mystery of Spirit.

We met one sunny autumn evening at a community drumming in a Grange Hall. For years, I had religiously driven two hours west from Port Townsend, to attend those monthly gatherings. It was there that I had first met Michael, who was to become a good friend, and his five-year-old daughter, Amy. While David had been a member of the men's movement for years, and knew Michael as a Lodge Brother, he had come that evening to this congregation of women, children and men, on the whim of an invitation.

At the outset of our courtship, David brought up the subject of his father. Of how he had promised to take care of him for the rest of his life, and to let him die at home. It dawned on me that the Cosmos was not only giving me, at fifty years of age, a husband and a marriage, it was also giving me another chance at having a father. I had no idea of what that would entail and even if I had, my starry-eyed romantic optimism simply would have embraced it all.

I first met Lincoln Brown, David's father, at Gwennie's Restaurant in Sequim, which served his all-time favorite breakfast of sausage gravy and biscuits. Because my work schedule allowed me an occasional flexible week day, I arrived soon after dawn on a sunny spring day, to find David's father eager to meet me.

Lincoln expected a kiss upon his cheek the moment David introduced us, for his son had spoken much of me and apparently "the sun rose and set" with me. Lincoln was a craggy old man with a thick head of hair, iron grey and silver, which the barber kept white-walled, and he was beardless. He and his son had much the same physique: broad of shoulder and deep of chest, powerful legs and beautiful hands. Lincoln's were gnarled, ancient and huge.

At that breakfast, as my beloved and I played footsies under the booth table and seduced each other with our eyes, Lincoln regaled me with stories of his many trades in life. He was a master storyteller with twinkles in his eyes, the hesitation of anticipation perfectly timed, and a sonorous voice which my beloved told me, had moved many a congregation. I was to hear those stories repeated over the coming years, even learned a few by heart.

Before I headed back to Port Townsend, I kissed Lincoln again, finding something comforting and connecting in kissing an old man's cheek. We were to exchange many, many such kisses in the future.

* * * * *

David's mother, Eva (née Knickenbocker) had been Lincoln's second wife, and their marriage had lasted more than forty years. Together as missionaries, they had taken their son traveling and preaching The Word all over the U.S, especially Alaska and the Four Corners Reservations of the Southwest. After retiring they had finally settled near Sequim, on the Olympic Peninsula, where the temperate seasons suited them.

David moved to be near them, and as the years unfolded his Mom became crippled with arthritis and high blood pressure. It was against her beliefs to take medications. So it was not surprising that, after David had just gotten home from spending the evening with his parents, his father called to say his mother had keeled over in the bathroom and was dead. Lincoln had already called 911. When David arrived, the paramedics were still working on her with no hope of resuscitation. Both men were appalled at the indignity of the paramedics' handling of their wife and mother, who had a massive cerebral hemorrhage and had gone to her Just Reward in a blink of an eye.

Although Lincoln was determined to remain independent, he was lost in his home without his wife. David was putting the finishing touches to a movie he had produced and had flown to California for a final conference. When he called to check up on his father. Lincoln was confused, very deaf and worried about his future. He told his son he thought he could no longer make it on his own.

As soon as David got back to town, he asked his father the only question needed: did he really want to live in a retirement home? Lincoln's reply was an emphatic no. So he came to live with his son, and worked with him in his antique refinishing business. Father and son started each day together with a hearty meal at Gwennie's.

Lincoln was still driving about in his beloved Old Blue pickup: going to church and taking out a widow from their socials, reading his Bible, allowing himself to watch "a little" television, and gardening. All this gave him a contented, interesting life.

When David's refinishing business prospered, he bought a split-level house overlooking the Straits, and moved Lincoln into his own basement apartment so he could continue his somewhat independent life. The State hired David to be his father's caregiver and take care of his finances, wellbeing and meals. Meanwhile David continued his Viet Nam Recovery work, facilitating Men's Groups and enjoying his Lodge brotherhood.

Their lives were full and busy.

*   *   *   *   *

I married David in my fiftieth year, and we were both hard at work. I moved to that split-level house in Sequim and commuted to Port Townsend, a lovely scenic hour's drive east, as I trained my successor at the doctor's practice where I had worked for more than nine years. On weekends, I helped father and son in their refinishing workshop.

It was all new and fascinating, this married life and these men.

We would work on the favored and antique pieces that customers shipped to us from all over the States. Lincoln stripped away the layers of varnish and paint on disassembled pieces which, when thoroughly cleaned and dried, David would refinish into a silky smoothness. Every

Monday, David and his father would travel around the community, answering queries received from their advertisement in the local newspaper.

One Saturday morning, in the summer of 1993, on his way to the workshop, Lincoln suddenly sat down on the steps outside his apartment. He could not tell us what was wrong, only that he felt dizzy and strange. We hurried him to the hospital in Port Angeles where they told us, after much testing, that he had suffered a mild stroke. On one of our visits to him, amid the forest of beeping and hissing machinery, Lincoln grabbed his son's hand, and made him promise that he would not allow him to die there. Once again David renewed his vow, and I stepped forward to make my own pledge.

A week later we brought Lincoln home. At first, because he was weak, we didn't think much about serving him his meals in his apartment. Then when we saw how arduous, even dangerous, climbing those stairs to come eat with us had become, we kept taking trays down to him. More and more, we saw less and less of him, and it didn't sit right with me. I was caught up in the busy-ness of the two magazines I managed, one of which I was handing off to my successor at the doctor's practice. The other, David and I ran from home. I couldn't think of a way to change any of it.

I hated knowing Lincoln was sitting all alone for hours, while we ran around like chickens without heads. It dawned on me that I hadn't got married for this. Day after day, David and I didn't see each other, other than at breakfast and as we headed for bed.

In the middle of one night, I awoke in a sweat (no, menopause was yet to come!), and sat at our dining table to write a long letter in which I enumerated what had changed, and how I thought to get out of the tar pit into which my husband and I had sunk.

I showed David the letter after I'd typed it up. Tears filled his eyes. Together we asked the Cosmos: what now? Now that this door was closing, what new ones were opening up for us?

That summer of 1993, the economy took a nosedive. Interest rates plummeted and by autumn, the financial backers for our magazine had melted away. By winter, no one was sending us their favored furniture for refinishing, and we realized that meeting the costs of that lovely house, and finding other work had became impossible. David and I, both hard workers who had always been able to make money, were faced with the realization that we could no longer support ourselves in the manner to which we'd become accustomed.

In the vows I had pledged to my husband was the one I had gladly given of taking care of his father's needs. We had been making friends, warily at first, because I was from big city life with no frames of references to his world of farming, church building, timber felling, mineral mining or missionary work. Yet we had like memories: he of the Depression and me of post-WWII England. We also shared a mischievous sense of humor.

When Lincoln came back from the hospital after that stroke, he was on a slew of new drugs. We began to notice that his abilities to stay in the present and to remember to do things, were becoming a danger. On the road in his beloved 1971 Chevrolet half ton pickup truck, which he had bought brand new, he would ignore traffic lights while taking his widow friend home, or forget his oil rag on the manifold while squiring me on errands. When his doctor revoked his driving privileges, it took so much out of him.

Then, his charming friend from church, whom he brought to Thanksgiving and Christmas feasts, was found dead in her home, and no one at the church thought to tell him about the funeral arrangements.

Lincoln was sinking into depression. His doctor's opinion, given in a hurried, unsympathetic moment during a visit, was: "Mr. Brown you're just growing old."

*   *   *   *   *

On a rainy winter day early in 1994, we were driving around the West End of the Olympic Peninsula, when we came upon a rare triangle acre of land for sale. It had a creek, access to electricity, and was beside a decently paved road. Within a month our bid had been accepted for that raw clear-cut property, where newly-sawn stumps of first growth hemlock and spruce reared up above the churned, devastated earth.

At home, in the workshop, we set about pre-building the frames to the homes we designed, and invited our friends out to help build Lincoln's eight-sided cabin.

Sometime during this hectic exodus, when we lived all day, every day together, planning and building, talking and eating, Lincoln became Poppa to me, became the father I'd not had as an adult, and he began to call me daughter.

Poppa, sitting under an umbrella in the rain, would supply the builders with screws, tools, steady hands, keen eyes and the wisdom of decades of building churches and homes. Most of my time was spent under a tarpaulin preparing huge feasts over portable propane rings with hauled in water, for our hungry crew.

Poppa seemed to rally with all the familiar things to do. He helped peel trees for the outhouse and woodshed, with tools he had used as a young man. As spring warmed the earth, he would bend over and fuss in our pathetic attempts to raise radishes, lettuces and beans in the dynamited and depleted earth. With no radio or television yet available in the valley, in the evenings he would read the books I found in our rural library about the pioneers of the area.

Meanwhile, we found a podiatrist to cut Poppa's distinctive toenails and monitor the health of his feet. We found a place to test his hearing and ordered hearing aids. On a drive by the Strait one day, Poppa mentioned that some men in a boat were in trouble because the tide was going out. We glanced at the water and saw three cormorants on a rock. We went looking for an eye doctor. We also discovered a miraculous chiropractor who brought much relief to his agéd sinews and bones.

Then we found a doctor in Forks who was skilled in geriatrics. He readily learned Poppa's particular way of describing his symptoms. This doctor had a sense of humor and was interested in his patients' lives and memories. When it was time for us to enter the exam room with Poppa, this doctor would come out to the waiting room to usher us in. I noticed he would watch the way Poppa walked. As he'd check out Poppa's vitals, the doctor would regale us with his fishing and hunting stories. He also knew how to speak to someone who was hard of hearing. In time he also became our doctor. Once he even stopped by our homestead on his way back from fishing on the lake. He wanted to show off his catch and took the opportunity to check Poppa's vitals. It seemed he always was interested in who we were and how we lived.

After a year, it was he who suggested Poppa get his knees replaced. The pain in Poppa's legs had become unbearable, making it out of bed was agony, and he was daily on painkillers. This doctor referred us to Virginia Mason, a teaching hospital in Seattle, renowned for its replacement surgery. After a daylong trip, Poppa was accepted into their program. Dr. Sorensen, the orthopedic surgeon, had asked him only one question: "Mr. Brown, why do you want your knees replaced at eighty-four years of age?" "If I can't walk, I might as well die." To which the good doctor had responded: "Well, you're not going to die, Mr. Brown, I'll replace your knees!"

Poppa would be his oldest patient. All the tests showed, however, that stroke notwithstanding, Poppa was an excellent candidate, in sound general health, with a powerful heart and good prospects for recovery.

I had knee surgery as a teenager, and I knew about physical therapy and willingly took Poppa's on. For that whole summer, it was our family's focus.

First, came the operation on Poppa's left knee, with David at his side in Seattle, and me taking care of the homestead. Quickly everyone learnt what drugs sent this Old Soul into bizarre hallucinations, and David was always there to bring him back. When Poppa got home, I again began his physical therapy regimen, and between us bloomed a sturdy relationship of Boss and Slave. We made many jokes and had a few spats. I was relentless, however, telling Poppa that the only pain he felt was that of his old other knee and the pain of the operation, which would soon fade.

Much to his amazement it did, and for the first time in years, Poppa felt no pain in his left leg.

In three months, he was eager for the next operation. By then I had his legs and arms strong and ready for the ordeal. Poppa also knew what to expect this time, and father and son set off for Seattle again.

The second convalescence occurred during the autumn and into a long wet winter, yet Poppa gladly braved the rain in his yellow slicker to walk the valley road. At first, only with me, as he learnt how his legs worked. Soon, he was on his own with his companion, Buddy-dog, on his leash. Buddy-dog, a totally black Labrador mix, had come to us as a yearling during the first summer we homesteaded. Now he was going on three years old. He had a loving disposition, a keen intelligence, was unusually modest about his business out on the land, and loved those walks along the road.

Poppa would always preface his walks with: "The doctor said walk or die!" And walk he did, rain or shine.

Poppa was thrilled to be pain-free, although once in a while he would hint that now more was expected of him. It was grand to see him get in and out of our minivan without a wince; step out of his cabin and walk over to ours for dinner, maneuvering our three steps with ease.

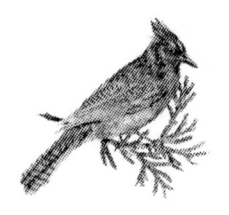

The Us of Us

Honoring our vows

"When do you think humans first discovered death?"
Bill Moyers, *The Power of Myth*

"In sickness and in health" was a phrase in my vows that began to roil around my mind. I had turned fifty when I became a wife, and went to live with a son whose father lived with him. An arrangement I thought not at all strange, even though we lived on the outskirts of Retirement Central, otherwise known as the Sequim Sunbelt.

Since the Greatest Generation finished raising their children, they had begun to retire, *en masse*, to this sunny, microclimate in the rain shadow of the Olympic Mountains. Developers had rushed in and bought out the original settlers' farms, and converted them into housing enclaves to which thousands of husbands and wives flocked. Many of the men had been wartime friends, while their wives had waited on the home front. They were the ones who tamed the raw developments with landscaping, bringing with them the fine furniture which we set about restoring.

We had lived on the fringes of a sprawling Western town that had found its vocation as a playground for those serious about learning to play again. Luxuriant golf courses were laid out surrounded by large, light-filled homes. Parklands were sculpted from potato and corn fields, complete with arched gateways and fetching names. The ratty hunters' and fishermen's RV parks got face lifts to accommodate all the prefabricated single and double-wide homes which started showing up in convoys on the backs of huge trailers, complete with pilot trucks flashing celebratory lights.

Churches and doctors abounded. Retirement apartment complexes and an aquatic exercise center were built. The marinas were expanded for all the year-round pleasure and fishing craft that came with the crowd, one of which was named after John Wayne, who had donated a nice parcel of land from his favorite Northwest retreat.

There sprung up a theater crowd, putting on lively performances, and the veterans' clubs prospered. The fishing and hunting were just dangerous and abundant enough, the weather enchanting, friends were plentiful and life was very good.

When the economy went south, and the denizens of Sequim hunkered down for some lean financial years, we moved on west to settle in a sparsely populated valley just ten miles from the Pacific Ocean. There we built our homes, reclaimed the devastated land, practiced our marriage and cared for our elder.

As Poppa progressed through his 80s, he enjoyed a pleasant and relaxing way of life. When the Cosmos sent us Buddy-dog, Poppa eagerly accepted the pup. Every day he walked the road with his companion, talked with neighbors, trained his dog, gardened with us, helped us plane lumber and, in the fall, went blackberry picking with me. He and Buddy-dog gladly joined us on trips to the seashore where we'd walk along the tide line, as I remembered doing with my father, along those distant English shores, during our summer holidays. Poppa and Buddy-dog were inseparable, and when Poppa joined us for dinner, he lay at Poppa's feet.

Once a month, we'd take a long day trip into Port Angeles for necessaries, a meal and occasionally, a movie. Every Sunday, I'd drive Poppa to his church, and for a short while, at the request of the church board, he had taught Sunday school. Now and again someone from church would bring him home.

In 1997, our doctor moved away to another practice, to be replaced by a young whipper-snapper who had never taken care of any elders. That year Poppa had been developing a series of unpleasant "heartburn" attacks. That's how he described them. His language about his body was sparse and vague. He knew in detail what lay under the hood of a pickup truck or any machine with a motor, yet he could hardly describe his insides and how they felt. *Just like the rest of us! I could tell you how a sewing machine worked or how to clean a vacuum cleaner. Could I describe how my pancreas worked or what an angina attack felt like?*

Soon, we were driving Poppa to this inexperienced doctor, twice a month as his systems began to seize up. Poppa was experiencing the bane of an old celibate man: the inability to whip it out in time. The doctor prescribed a mind-boggling, ever-changing array of pills, some with horrible side effects. With Poppa's herniated esophageal valve, aggravated by his stomach being compressed by his bent spine, the result of handling his father's horse-drawn plow, vomiting was dangerous. When aspiration occurred into his lungs, he would gasp and cough, wheeze and become dizzy. Other drugs took away his appetite, made him confused and weak.

Meanwhile, Poppa was also on a handful of drugs for stroke prevention, digestion and blood thinning. His daily regimens of pills morning, noon and evening were a constant irritation to us all. In part because he resisted taking them, as it meant he had to drink water, which meant he'd have to pee. In part because there were so many, and some of them were dangerous if taken too close together.

For two more years, we struggled in ignorance as Poppa's health and *joie de vivre* faltered. *What was going wrong?* Was Poppa simply too tired from nearly nine decades of life? Was his warranty finally running out? Had the knee surgery over-stressed him? The trade off was he had long ago quit needing painkillers.

A typical day at the doctor's would begin with a wake up that could vary from lively to lethargic. While David prepared breakfast, I would be over at Poppa's helping him with his morning rituals. We'd hang around long enough for Poppa to have a bowel movement, eat breakfast and get ready to go.

Usually we had to wait for the doctor, so Poppa, Buddy-dog and I would walk outside in slow measured circuits around the clinic, looking at the new landscape and letting Buddy-dog sniff in all the new places. When we'd be called in for his check up, the doctor, more often than not, would find nothing new and simply order a blood draw. We would walk Poppa across to the hospital lab where Chauncey, the sure-handed vampire, would joke with us as he drew blood.

Then we'd be off to the supermarket for supplies, a good walk for Poppa as he pushed the shopping cart, and picked out his favorite candy bars and fruit. Often we'd stop at the pharmacy for a new prescription. Usually we'd take our dinner at a loggers' restaurant where we'd all eat heartily. When the weather was dry, we'd make a picnic somewhere where Buddy-dog could have a good time too. Then we'd make the pleasant highway drive home through forest and beside lakes.

For years we had been insisting Poppa drink three pint bottles of well water every day. If he had his way, the only time he'd have drunk water was with his pills. It didn't matter that without water his system dried up, BMs didn't happen, and he'd feel miserable as the toxins backed up, prunes and stool softeners notwithstanding.

Every time Poppa refused a water bottle, I'd clearly hear Jo Hyde-Smith's voice ringing in my head. During my last visit back to England, my daughter and I had stayed over at Jo's home on the Suffolk coast. One evening, we had taken her out for a posh dinner at the local inn. There, we Americans had to request glasses of water from a surprised waiter. While we quaffed as if there was a drought, Jo, wine glass in hand, had snorted: "Never touch the stuff!" I think Poppa felt the same way!

We found that when we did condom catheter Poppa at night he would rip it off (*Ouch! He would say he hadn't felt a thing!*) trying to get to a urinal bottle. The small daytime bags meant we had to empty them every two hours, day or night. We learnt that those bags didn't have a back-up valve, when one night Poppa forgot he was cathetered, and successfully tore off the tubing, and the urine had drained away onto the bed and floor. If he didn't drink water, he wouldn't poop which made him miserable. The irony was, that when he didn't drink he didn't have to worry about peeing. Daytime condom cathetering allowed him to sit for hours without moving which he preferred, and worked well when we were on a trip.

Years before, I had cut off the guard flaps in his long johns, which he wore all the time. There was nothing we could do with his trousers. I once wondered about inventing a Velcro-type fly, and quickly realized it would probably amount to the same fumbling with numb fingers. Besides those little hooks could scratch up such tender flesh!

And then the Summer of 1999 turned into Fall, and the month of October became a watershed in Poppa's health. Scary symptoms came and went; came and stayed, and this valiant Old Soul began fading fast. No amount of pills or combinations of them nor clinic visits seemed to change anything. Unable to explain or diminish the recurring symptoms of vomiting, tiredness and dizziness, our trust and confidence in the doctor's abilities sank.

The days grew more and more littered with distress. "Heartburn" would flare up at odd moments, sometimes relieved by antacids and water, sometimes with a liquid analgesic, and sometimes they simply had to be ridden through. During one such attack, David thought to pop one of the old nitroglycerin pills, prescribed by the earlier doctor, under Poppa's tongue, and we waited.

Surprisingly swiftly, Poppa felt relief. We watched him uncurl, watched the grimace of pain leave his face. Then came an astonishing headache which, just as suddenly, subsided. David rushed to the telephone to tell the doctor, instead he had to leave a message with the answering service.

A week later we were at the clinic again and the doctor, when we told him we had given Poppa some more nitro pills when other attacks had occurred, agreed that Poppa's "heartburn" had nothing to do with his stomach and everything to do with his heart. The doctor ordered us to quit one set of pills, start another, gave us a fresh prescription for the nitro pills, and sent us home.

I began learning about pain relief: about having to mash up "horse" pills because Poppa was gagging on them, how long those pills took to work, and how the nitro pills gave him a huge headache. *Isn't there a liquid form? A patch?*

The next Sunday, on my Godliness-next-to-Cleanliness day, Poppa threw up an hour after he'd taken a newly prescribed pill. He hadn't had breakfast yet, so there wasn't anything other than prunes, pills and water to come up. I was frantic. *What's with this vomiting?* He's so miserable and apologetic.

"It's all right, Poppa, don't worry about it. I wish I could do something to stop it." *Of course it's not all right! What does this vomiting mean?* When we do get through to him, the doc's no help. Try this pill, change these, stop that one.

In time, Poppa asked for breakfast, and then said he still wanted to go to church. As we cruised through the hilly timber farms, he was alert and spoke to Buddy-dog. I helped him into the chapel, reminded him about his nitro pills, and sped off to do the laundry, get the mail, pick up some shopping, and take a walk on the beach with Buddy-dog.

When I was done, I waited in the church parking lot. Soon everyone was pouring out of the chapel. No Poppa. I went in and found him sleepily sitting in a pew. I helped him back to the car. He was so tired. I checked his catheter bag, hardly anything in it. No, he hadn't had to use any nitro pills. *Strange how no one at the church helps him out of the chapel.*

As we drove home he perked up and eagerly ate his snack of half a cheese sandwich with a cut up apple, all the while sucking up through a straw, one of those nutrition-rich drinks.

There we were driving along, chatting and enjoying the ride, when suddenly the pain attacked. I stopped in a turnout and opened Poppa's door, found the bottle of nitro pills in his pocket, and popped one in under his tongue. Poppa leaned back and waited for the relief. In five minutes, he grunted "About 20% relief." I gave him a second pill and we waited. Near 50% now. The instructions were that he could have three in a row at five minute intervals. That day was the first of many three pill attacks.

We hurried home to tell David.

It took the whole month for us to quit denying that something was wrong, to realize that no amount of exercise, good food and loving care was going to turn his health around.

It took all of this month, with two emergency hospital visits, for the doctor to realize that his oldest patient was in trouble.

All through that month I was shocked at how ignorant I was about the way a body stopped working. How a mind ceased to think.

Each episode of pain came on at different times, especially in the night, keeping us awake with worry and wonder. People we met began telling us about long-term care homes that would know what to do and how to care for him. They queried us about why we kept Poppa home, and hinted that perhaps we didn't know what we were doing or what we were in for. Sometimes, I wondered too!

One day Poppa woke up befuddled and white-faced. David and I were with him constantly that day. After a nap in his chair, Poppa wanted up so I gave him his canes. He started to stand and keeled over. I caught him and let him rest on the floor until he could get up. Immediately he needed to pee and I brought him a urinal. We had been asking the doctor for condoms catheters and bags, and all the gear that goes with them: hoses, sterile water, swabs, etc. As if it's not undignified enough that he can't whip it out in time, now he had to beg for the things he needed to continue to function in modesty! We had to beg! *Why is there no strength in Poppa's legs? Why is he so pale, so confused and dizzy?*

Walking with Poppa had ground down to a snail's pace. Jokingly, he would mutter that the slugs outran him! Such gruff humor deserved a hug and a kiss and he would pat my hand, shyly glancing up at me and tell me he loved me too, and on we'd plod in the cool October air.

More often than not, Poppa would make it to his porch each day and set up residence in his chair. If he sat still, the chipmunks would venture up to him, foraging for the seeds he slowly dribbled down his trouser leg to the floor. Frequently I would hear Poppa's version of a giggle as a critter would scamper up his leg and then, in shock, hightail it down.

For someone who loved his food, suddenly he was pushing away his plate and groaning as the pain enveloped him and once it had subsided, he'd have no appetite. We began to serve him light snacks several times a day.

Some mornings, Poppa would wake on his own and set about his chores, forget where he was in the ritual and end up asleep again. Sometimes he would sit on the side of his bed, conscious and talking about how he wanted to shave, what he wanted for breakfast and how, later, he'd like to take a walk. Some mornings he was silent, glassy-eyed and unresponsive as if his body was just too heavy to cart around anymore, letting me dress him and shoo him to his recliner.

Some nights, the alarm would ring in our bedroom, and we'd find him confused and flailing with the pain and we'd tend to him, one of us napping in his recliner until he was without pain and asleep again.

Halfway through October, we trundled over to Poppa's in the middle of the night in answer to the alarm, to find him wheezing mightily. He said it reminded him of childhood asthma attacks. Listening to his breathing in the stethoscopic, sounded like Velcro being opened. His nose was running and he was coughing. *What was this?* We called the hospital nurses' station and were told to watch for lessening or worsening of symptoms. His doctor was not on call, so another one had to field this episode blind.

When, three hours later, there was no subsidence of the symptoms, we called the nurses' station again and their reaction was: "Bring him in!" We bundled him warmly with Buddy-dog beside him, and drove the hour to Forks along the empty dark roads. It has ever been our practice, since moving out here, to keep our gas tank at least half full because after 10pm there are no gas stations open.

That first hospitalization was traumatic for us all. The separation showed us just how disconnected Poppa had become. He couldn't hear the nurses or the TV; couldn't remember the rituals they expected of him; couldn't find the call button on his bed, hated the oxygen pipes in his nose, hated the tasteless food. No salt or pepper allowed!

Once his symptoms had diminished, the doctor released him back to our care, at last giving us the Rxs for 24 hours a day condom catheters. He also told us to prepare for a visit to Seattle for further cardiac testing. When we got home, David began long hours on the telephone working out the arrangements with ParaTransit and Virginia Mason. While Poppa had been in the hospital, he had been hooked up to an oxygen tube. We were sent home without any, *why?*

The episodes of pain increased. The nurses' station told us to do this and do that, change these meds, give those pills, raise him, keep him warm, and to watch for sweating and any change in color.

David collected a donated, old hospital bed from the defunct Forks Hospice. *How could a town, full of elders, not have use for a Hospice Center?*

Then came the night when the nitro didn't work. Poppa had a relentless pain and was wheezing heavily. Still we had no oxygen. We stayed with him for hours until at last, the night nurse told us to dial 911. Within minutes Ed Wilbur, who lived a mile along the road, arrived with a bottle of oxygen and a two-way radio. He immediately clamped the oxygen mask on Poppa's pale face, and set about checking Poppa's vitals. Then he called for an ambulance.

Forty-five minutes later, with flashing lights, the ambulance backed up our driveway, and out leapt friends and fellow congregants of Poppa. Glen, the driver, had brought Poppa home from church a time or two. With much gruff greetings, the paramedics bundled him onto the gurney and hurtled off into the night.

At four o'clock in the morning, we were left standing, in a rare star and moonlit night, listening to the chorus of Buddy-dog's barking and coyotes' yipping.

In that special moment David and I spoke of the life and death things we have to say to know how we're feeling, where we might be going and how best we may be of service. David worried about wrong and right actions, and I worried about nasty and nice emotions. Husband and wife, yin and yang.

Once again the empty days of tidying up Poppa's cabin and organizing supplies, of driving to the hospital for visits and conferences with the doctor. *He doesn't know squat! Got the feeling he's going to chalk this one up to "practicing" his profession.* Never did learn to communicate with Poppa; always looked at us askance, as if we were bugs from another planet, and now he doesn't know what's the matter. *Damn! I wish that other doc had stayed!*

Home to telephone Poppa's far-flung relatives.

Early the next morning, the doctor called. Lincoln had another bad night of pain and wheezing right there in the hospital. *Why? Doesn't know. So it's not our primitive nursing skills and/or lifestyle!* The doctor has ordered an ambulance to transport Poppa to Virginia Mason in Seattle, so we'd better get ourselves there!

When we arrived at the hospital, Poppa was anxious, confused and very deaf, repeatedly appealing to David to go with him to Seattle.

As the staff began prepping Poppa for the ride, I got my goodbyes in. Then I handed-off our minivan so David could follow the ambulance, and be at his father's side when the doctors had to speak to Poppa, letting him know what they had planned for him.

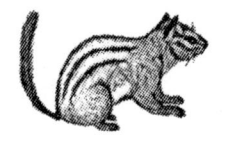

Day 1

Our paths into The Valley

*"...the troubles of my heart are enlarged
O bring thou me out of my distress."*

Psalm 25

For five days, I have lived alone on our homestead out in the timber farms and rainforest of the Olympic Peninsula, without my husband and father-in-law at my side. Five nights of sleeping alone with Buddy-dog creeping from his blankets to lie quietly at the foot of our bed.

Over the past year Poppa's health has deteriorated with daily episodes of "heartburn" and vomiting. We have had to watch him become more and more weary, short of breath, dizzy and disoriented while being ordered to give him a tonic, and an assortment of stomach pills with unpleasant side-effects. He has been in the local hospital twice already this month and has now been transported via ambulance to Virginia Mason Hospital in Seattle for observation and testing. Poppa's primary care physician's final opinion before signing off on his oldest patient was, "It's congestive heart failure, Mr. Brown. Your father has a 50/50 chance of making it to surgery, less than 50/50 of making it through and less than 50/50 chance of making a full recovery."

My husband is at his father's side and I have been waiting at home, preparing Poppa's cabin for his return, praying that by that very cleaning, he *will* return. Five days with one miserably lost Buddy-dog. Our neighbors have willingly helped when I needed it. I have been holding safe and sacred space for this beloved Old Soul and his son as they traverse this next plateau together.

Before Poppa was moved into the ambulance that would take him on the five-hour trip east, I gave him my love and thanks for supporting us all these years, both financially and with the vastness of his skills as we cleared and built our homestead upon this newly logged land. All we have planned and completed here, has the wisdom and knowledge gleaned from Poppa's stroke-stricken mind.

For five sunny autumn days, I have been waiting, putting up the garden for winter, splitting and hauling wood, bringing in water and cooking meals for one. Five days of neighbors calling for news and bringing our mail out to me, of writing in my journal and walking along the road with a confused Buddy-dog.

Etched new and raw are the scenes of Poppa in distress. At home, and at the Forks hospital where his doctor decided to send him to the mainland specialists. At Poppa's insistence, David had made a call to Poppa's pastor. "Please come, Lincoln has asked for some spiritual solace."

Memories of Poppa hanging onto his son's hand as they bundled him in blankets onto a gurney. I too was holding his hand, kissing his cheek and telling him I loved him and, just before he was wheeled out to the waiting ambulance, he called my name and told me he loved me.

Still no pastor.

Memories of gripping my husband's hand, leaning close to his comforting bulk, talking of all the things he'd have to remember alone there in the big city. Would he remember his own pills and needs? So used now was he to living in tandem with me, would he take care of himself as well as his father?

When I called good neighbor Bob Johnson to ask the favor that he drive all the way to Forks to pick up Buddy-dog and me and bring us home, I was relieved to hear his immediate: "Setting out right now!" In an hour he would arrive. In an hour David, would be rounding Crescent Lake in the wake of the ambulance, on his way to Seattle, affectionately known as the Emerald City.

After reluctant kisses and hugs, I was left standing alone in the pouring rain with Buddy-dog on his leash. We watched, as husband and master drove away after his father, and then we waited. To relieve the worry, we walked around the hospital block. As we walked and waited, I found myself remembering my best friend MerryJo.

For twelve years MerryJo's and my lives had mingled as we worked in a domestic violence prevention program, and raised our children together. Then I got a call from MerryJo's oldest daughter that her mother was dying over at VMH.

David and I had sped across the Peninsula to get there in time. As we slid to a stop in the ferry parking lot, the ferry was just pulling away. I burst into tears. The loading guard, who knew me from the domestic violence program, poked her head into our window: "What's wrong?" When I told her, she used her two-way radio to call the ferry back. The big ship stopped in the water, and then quickly backed up. The ramp was lowered, and our minivan was squeezed on board. I cried all the way over, while David took a nap.

When we walked into the ICU, a hectic and disjointed vigil was in progress, with MerryJo's daughters in hysterics. While their mother had been slowly ailing, her dying had come suddenly. The ICU was filled with machines and nurses, doctors and friends all stark and cold under harsh glaring lights. Noise filled the air as a breathing machine hummed and gushed, while others beeped and burped. Everyone was in a high state of anxiety, pacing and squatting against walls.

I had waded through the throng to kiss my friend's forehead, and murmur in her ear that I loved her. Beneath the mask that flattened her face into an unkind grimace, she seemed to be in an uneasy sleep. The breathing machine forced her chest to rise and fall, and her bare arms were covered with tape and tubes. I stroked her unkempt grey hair, and looked long upon the face of my friend, gaunt now, with such a fragile pallor. As I smoothed her hair down, I thanked her for her years of support and friendship. Memories of the many good times we had shared, flitted across my mind.

Soon, other friends arrived, and I was shuffled off to the side.

For a few hours, David and I lingered in that crazy atmosphere of weeping women and silent men. MerryJo's pastor went from person to person, speaking words of spiritual comfort, offering prayers.

A week later, at the formal funeral service in which my friend's name was mentioned only once, I was uncomfortable with the impersonal and scripted ceremony. Instead of a personal farewell, where her friends and loved-ones spoke of their joy of knowing MerryJo; spoke of what a difference this brave and true woman had made in their lives, everyone was moping about in timid misery.

When the organist began playing the hymns MerryJo had so loved, I was not surprised to hear no one singing. I, who was not a church member and hadn't sung those songs since my Church of England school years, stood up and sang my heart out for my friend's repose.

Afterwards, I took out my Spirit Drum and sang my friend's songs as the mourners filed out of that little church into the bright June sunshine. When I was done, the pastor surprised me by coming over to thank me.

Had I been a drinker, I'd have gone to the nearest bar and raised a glass of MerryJo's favorite beverage, a Tom Collins, to her memory. Instead I sang her my spirit songs.

I dreaded the thought of Poppa dying over at Virginia Mason like my friend. I prayed that they would stabilize him and send him home where he belonged. And so I walked around in the rain, until Bob's pickup rolled into the drenched parking lot and Buddy-dog and I clambered aboard.

Still no pastor.

As Bob drove home, I let the soggy autumn landscape flood by me, and I wearily pondered on what could have been more important on a Saturday afternoon, than for a pastor to administer spiritual solace to one of his flock.

By that evening David had called with the first diagnosis: congestive heart failure. The specialists at Virginia Mason were astonished at the deterioration of Poppa's heart and at the inexpert prescribing of drugs.

For five days, I kept the home fires burning and waited. David's phone calls were bright oases in the long days alone.

At some point David was advised to set up a hospital bed in Poppa's cabin and we decided I had better get the hospice donated bed out of our ancient pickup Bessie, and into place. With the help of Bob, Emil Person and his son

Stephen, we dragged that heavy metal machine over our gravel paths and through Poppa's door. With much huffing and puffing the deed was done, and my kindly neighbors departed. I was left waiting again, making up the old bed and plugging it in to see what the buttons did, the icons were so faded they gave no indication. All seemed to work, and I continued about my busy-ness, readying Poppa's cabin.

Suddenly I heard a motor start up and turning around, watched this empty bed raise and lower itself. Later as I was showering, I heard the motor again. After drying off, I came out to find the bed head in its upright position. As I stared, of its own accord, it lowered itself again!

By the third day of waiting, I had begun asking people about the steps to the Dance of Death. *Who do we contact? Who has to know, and when? What are the laws in this state concerning dying at home? Are there home nursing agencies and who would know about them? Ah, yes!* We went to a conference last year and got a handful of pamphlets from various companies, they should be in Poppa's file. *How do we choose?*

A funeral home in the county seat, Port Angeles, finally, without coyness or pseudo-religious euphemisms, began answering my questions beyond: "Call us, that's what we're here for. We'll take care of everything." One salesman came striding across our land a day later, all dressed up in his camouflage, reminding me it was hunting season. He offered me a folder filled with business cards, instructions and forms.

I wanted to know the steps ahead of time, for there would be no dress rehearsal. This was a once in a lifetime occasion, and I wanted to know how society expected it done.

I had come to think of getting ready for death as similar to preparing for a child's birth. Except there are no midwives should you choose to have a home death. I wanted to know what must we do when we found Poppa dead in his bed. Who knew and who answered, was a revelation.

Not Poppa's pastor. I had interrupted him at a church meeting, and could hear voices in the background yelling instructions, one of which was: "Call 911, we need to practice our resuscitation techniques!"

Not Poppa's doctor. I had miraculously been connected between appointments. "I don't know, Rebecca, ask the police." We're so rural we don't have our own police, only a County Sheriff and the State Patrol, all over an hour's drive away.

Not the hospital. Neither the receptionist nor the nurses' station knew what to do with a home death. "Not here, call the funeral home you booked."

Each person's tone of voice implied, "wouldn't everyone rather die in a hospital?"

It was Wednesday, October 27, when David called me to tell me of the doctor's prognosis, that Poppa had no more than three months to live, and that he had decided to come home to die. Father and son would be setting out the next morning. As my husband and I said goodbye, we spoke of how today had been Day One of Standing The Watch.

Thursday, as David and Poppa were driving home, a huge truck rumbled up our driveway, a chap leapt out of the cab, clipboard in hand and greeted Buddy-dog with enthusiasm. He was from a medical supply company in Port Angeles, and had been instructed by Virginia Mason Hospital to bring out an oxygen compressor and kit. He wrestled a large machine out from the side of his truck, and hooking it up to the tank on the back, flipped a switch. As the roaring machine did its thing, he chatted with me about the Hoko elk herd, the health of the deer population, and the differences between city and country living. Soon the roaring ceased. He said he was ready to start moving stuff into place. The gravel paths, which David and I had taken weeks to lay down so Poppa and I had smooth, mud-free surfaces to walk along, were now proving a hindrance to rolling wheeled things.

When we got into Poppa's cabin, he stood thinking. Not enough room. Where best to set the compressor as far away from the wood stove as possible? Poppa's cabin is round, with every wall occupied by shelves, windows and clothes racks.

The huge old hospital bed was stuck out from the west wall, so in beside it went the compressor, and then I received a fast course on oxygen. When the chap turned on the machine, the whole cabin throbbed and was filled with noise. *No one is going to like this!* A new word came into my reality: cannula, the tubing that would go into Poppa's nose, piping in the oxygen.

How I wished I was not alone as he bid goodbye and hoisted himself into the cab. Buddy-dog followed the truck to the end of the drive and sat there waiting. How lost we both have been, waiting for our family to come home.

David's drive into The Valley

These are David's memories of that grey October day, when we were told that Poppa had to go to Seattle to see a specialist. They seem lit by spotlights on unconnected scenes.

"*I remember the midnight awakening to Poppa's alarm, his labored breathing; giving the nitro tabs; calling 911 and speaking with Ed Wilbur, our neighbor and one-and-only* local EMT along the road, and when he arrived, him giving Poppa oxygen. I took some heart as color came back into that grey old face and his breathing eased. I felt an utter helplessness, unable to affect events and feeling pulled by an inexorable tide into depths where I didn't know how to swim.

In some part of my psyche was growing an understanding that my father was dying. On the periphery of this maelstrom I felt as a little boy, crying and clenching his fists, saying, over and over again: "No! No! No!"

It was raining as the ambulance backed into the driveway, and Poppa's little cabin became crowded with people, emergency gear and gurney. I remember standing in the rain watching the MedUnit, with its bright lights, pulling away into the darkness, headed for Forks. Because I had taken my meds for the diabetic neuropathy that plagued my legs, I couldn't follow and I was awash with helplessness as that ambulance took my father.

Six hours later, we got to Forks, and walked into Poppa's hospital room, the same one he'd been in before. I saw his own helplessness mirrored back at me.

"Sorry to be such a burden to you, Son." My father wheezed as I held his hand.

"Well, let's see, Poppa. You took care of me for eighteen years and I've taken care of you for thirteen. I think there's still a credit in your favor!" It was good to see him smile.

Waiting for the doctor, waiting for the doctor, waiting.

At some time the doc told us he was sending Poppa on to Seattle's Virginia Mason Hospital for tests and the care of a cardiologist. He murmured phrases about valve replacements, probability of success, etc., etc., etc.

I remember Poppa asking me if I would call his pastor who lived thirteen miles away to request he come administer to

Poppa. On reaching the pastor, I heard his hesitation, and then I was caught up again in the hurry up and wait at the hospital until, two hours later, as Poppa was being bundled into the ambulance, I realized the pastor had never turned up.

As my wife and I walked through the rain to our minivan in the parking lot, we talked about what we were going to do. I was torn about leaving her alone and having to follow my father. The ambulance wouldn't wait for us, so we hurriedly hugged and kissed goodbye. I started up the van and followed the diminishing tail lights of the ambulance as it headed east to the mainland, on a trip that I had no idea how it was going to end.

I remember following that ambulance, seemed like an experience out of a book I had read: losing it in traffic; pushing our little four cylinder van as hard as it could go to catch up; going over hills and down the other side; catching sight again of the ambulance; catching up. Thinking I knew where it was going, it would suddenly turn off on roads I'd never traveled before, taking a route to what I hoped was the ferry at Bainbridge Island.

With its lights flashing, the ambulance went straight to the ferry, not even slowing down for the toll booth or the parking lot. The flaggers stopped me and I had to explain I was following my father and then they waved me on.

On the ferry I sat in the ambulance, holding Poppa's hand and talking with the Medics all the way over the water, the beep of the heart machine in rhythm with the ferry's motor. I listened with dread to the rasping sound of my father's breathing in the oxygen mask. Holding a hand that was so cold.

I remember arriving at Virginia Mason Hospital, looking for a place to park in the dark and hurrying to the emergency room; being told Poppa had already been sent on to the 8th Floor Cardiac Unit, and getting there to wait, always the waiting, while they made Poppa comfortable, stabilized, IDed him and got him drugged.

There was no place for me to lie down or rest my legs. Always the sitting and the waiting in utter helplessness, not even able to read the book I'd brought along. I walked the hospital corridors at four in the morning because I could no longer stand to sit in a chair. When I found a couch in a waiting room where people lingered for their friends and loved-ones to come out of surgery, I laid down and slept for an hour. Then I awoke and trudged back to Poppa's room, waiting for something to happen. By then, my legs were on fire all the time.

I vaguely remember doctors in white coats coming in and talking to Poppa and me; taking notes, nodding their heads as if what we said made sense in a world that had no sense. Poppa being taken for an echocardiogram and waiting for someone to tell us the results. The dread when we were told that he was getting less than 15% pressure out of his left ventricle. Four years ago, when Poppa had his knees replaced here, the heart specialist had said his heart was pumping at 50-60%, the heart capacity of a man thirty years younger.

One day, I remember being awakened, after having fallen asleep in the chair next to Poppa's bed, by the murmur of voices and seeing the cardiologist with his train of attendant residents, telling how Poppa was going to have an angiogram, and then the waiting. That afternoon they took him away. Again I waited. In time, they wheeled Poppa back in, with his legs cushioned in air bags with pressure cuffs pumping rhythmically to keep the blood in his legs from clotting. How haggard and white was my father's face. That night the doctor made his rounds and had no answers. More waiting.

Sometime during daylight I made contact with the hospital's social services, explaining the situation: the distance from home; the lack of support we had in this huge city. As if by magic, after a hurried conference with the floor nurses, Poppa was moved to another room and a rollaway cot was brought in. That night, for the first time, I was able to stretch out with my clothes off and sleep for six hours straight. I awoke to the bustle of nurses and aides. I showered and pulled on the same old clothes and waited again.

Later the cardiologist showed up to discuss Poppa's condition. Time at that point seemed to have no meaning. Even though I was wearing a watch again for the first time in years, I could never seem to remember to look at it or fit it into my references about what was happening or when it happened.

Another spotlight with no reference point to time, is of me standing beside my father's bed with him half raised, oxygen tubes stuck in his nose. I was looking at a doctor who seemed to float in a very real manner in a very unreal situation, listening to the words that came out of his mouth. He seemed to take on substance and then vanish into thin air.

"Your heart's wore out, Mr. Brown. It's like an old tire. I could put in a new valve but I can't patch the tire because it's so thin and worn. Putting in a new valve might blow out the sidewalls." I remember thinking how that explanation was so clear and in a language that Poppa could understand. It was an incredibly relieving moment.

"If I put you on the table, Mr. Brown, in my experience, I don't think you would survive the operation. Even if you did survive, you'd have to go to a long-term facility for at least six months for recuperation. So the decision is yours."

Poppa and I had looked at each other, understanding everything that had been said, and at the same time refusing to comprehend.

"Without the operation, how long do you think he has?"

The doctor answered without hesitation, "No more than three months, Mr. Brown, no more than three months!" I remember staring at that doctor willfully, unable to turn my head and look at my father.

"What is your recommendation?"

And the doctor, looking not at me but at Poppa answered, "I really don't want to do this operation. I don't think you can survive it. Please don't make me take my knife to you, Mr. Brown, but the decision has to be yours."

I finally turned to Poppa, realizing he was not looking at the doctor but at me: "What do you want to do, Dad?"

"I want to go home, Son! I want to go home and I want to watch the blue jays. You promised me, Son. You promised I wouldn't die in a hospital." I could feel his urgency as his hand reached out and grasped mine.

I remember the feel of tears on my cheeks, suddenly released and flowing down into my beard, hot and then cold. The moment was completely empty of time, like standing amidst a glade in the forest completely surrounded, isolated, no forward, no back, no comprehension of how I got there, no comprehension of where I was going.

"Yes, I did, Poppa." And with those words, I knew that time was once again on the march, moving forward. Now the first steps of the journey to a destination lay before us.

There was a sigh, and I realized it wasn't me or Poppa. Turning my head I met the eyes of that eminent thoracic surgeon who seemed only to have enough breath to say, "Thank you, Mr. Brown, I think you've made the absolute best decision you could ever make! Thank you!"

I became aware suddenly of where I really was and the feel of Poppa's hand in mine, waiting for me to take the lead, as I had done so many times, to set off down this path we had chosen to walk thirteen years before when he'd come to live with me after Mom died.

I remember a hurried conversation about discharge, oxygen companies, home health care services and medications. Because of our long journey, he would be discharged the next day, Thursday. And then everybody was gone from the room leaving Poppa and me waiting.

As Poppa lay there quietly, I called Rebecca to tell her the news. I remember the tears coming again as I told her of Poppa's wish to come home. And that once again, I had reaffirmed to my father, that he could die at home.

I told my wife that I felt like I was starting a Guard Watch for Poppa, and that today had been the First Day of that Watch.

That night Poppa had pain and hallucinations; he was convinced his beloved pickup truck, Old Blue, was waiting down on the street and how we had to get to it because we had a long drive ahead. Little did I know the drive would not be that long.

Morning came with some clarity to his agéd mind as the nurses prepped, escorted and loaded Poppa for departure. I pulled out of the loading zone, headed up Pill Hill where all the hospitals in Seattle seemed to have clustered, around the corner and on down to the waiting ferry.

In the hustle and bustle of that wake up, I had condom catheterered and bagged Poppa, and he sat in the passenger seat exhausted, his head back against the headrest, seemingly floating between here and there.

The journey was mostly silent until we got close to Sequim, when Poppa asked if we could go by Mom's grave. I pulled into the little country cemetery, jouncing and bouncing across the pot holes, trundling around to the backside where we could see her headstone and we just sat there with the unspoken realization between us that he would soon join her in this little plot of earth looking up at the Olympic Mountains.

Neither of us could move. We just sat until finally, in a surprisingly strong voice, Poppa broke the silence. "All right, Son, let's go home!"

We arrived home in a golden sunset and, as I honked the horn, out rushed Rebecca with grins of greeting and Buddy-dog silently leaping and prancing in circles as we unloaded, getting Poppa as far as his recliner in his cabin.

It was so good to be back, and yet it felt so bad!

I remember a feeling of incomprehensible stillness as I stood in Poppa's cabin looking out at the picnic table that Rebecca had pulled up right in front of the window and realized that I was watching a chipmunk in late October, gleaning the seeds and dancing around an indignant blue jay. Poppa sat in his chair, craning his neck to see his critters, with a big smile on his face.

Now we had started The Walk into The Valley of Death and there would be no more stops along the way. Little did I know that it wouldn't be three months, but only thirteen days of Standing The Watch, and that this had been Day Two."

* * * * *

Dear Cyber Friends,

Your emails give me much comfort, please keep chatting to me, it makes me feel so good. It's interesting who has not responded to my emails about Poppa. I guess dying is a bit of a *faux-pas* in some people's lives, eh? Stay close to me.

I'm making cottage pie for my men as they tool in across the Peninsula and then David will need to sleep and sleep and sleep, as I'm sure the neuropathy in his legs is really bad for not having enough rest at night. Once he's taught me what I need to learn about the new level of care for the Poppadum, he can collapse into his wonderful bed and sleep.

Other than that? My stress rash is in full bloom. I've no appetite although I've enjoyed cooking with herbs and eating little meals. I hope I can keep it up when they get back. I expect both of them have dropped in weight. Poppa's appetite has slowly come back, although early this morning, David remarked that it was as if he'd given up. Poppa wouldn't talk, eat, look at you or respond. Then when David called from the ferry dock, Poppa was chipper again and eating, go figure!

I love you. Let me chat at you like this and you chat back. xoxRebeccaxox

Log excerpt for Day Three of The Watch

Friday, October 29 First morning home.
07:00am A good night! Poppa wide awake & hungry: "Good morning, Sweetheart, what's for breakfast?" Catheter held all night. Urine bag 800cc bright yellow. Drank entire Rx beverage. Ate half his breakfast.
09:15 Gave him his morning meds + 200cc water.
10:30 Insisted on a shower & shave "...to get the big city hospital off of me!" Wanted to get fully dressed. David re-cathetered him so he could sit in his recliner "...like a normal human being!"
11:15 Home health nurse arrived to take vitals.
Noon Enjoyed a bowl of soup+crackers+Rx drink. Walked on his own to his porch seat & looked out at the land. Chipmunks still here! *Amazing!*
03:40 Wanted to come over to our cabin for dinner. Ate as if he were starved: "Good enough to make a young coyote sit up and sass his grandma!" Enjoyed catching up with the local paper. Helped him back for a nap. Emptied catheter bag.
05:00 Woke him for meds. Really tired. Didn't want to watch TV, just wanted to go to bed.
06:10 On his bed, in his pjs, he had pain. Gave 1 nitro tab.
06:20 Pain reduced 65%.
06:30 Pain almost gone. Laid back & dozed off.
09:05 Woke with a groan. Sharp bad pain w/grimace. Heavy breathing. 1 nitro + calming pill. Held his hands while waiting. *This is going to take some getting used to!*
09:12 No change. l more nitro. Pain severe. *I hate this*!

09:17 1 more nitro. *Please, give him some relief!*

09:22 Pain reduced "...quite a bit." Nearly 50%. Nitro headache.

09:50 Still 50% or more pain. BP49/34. Talked to the home health nurse: lie Poppa flat & elevate his legs. Poppa cannot swallow these huge pills; the nurse told us how to crush up a pain relief cocktail. *This is absurd!*

10:30 BP127/75. Just "a little bit" of pain left. Breathing heavy.

11:05 Comfortable. No pain. Very sleepy. *Who isn't!*

01:50am Sleeping & snoring.

Soon so will we!

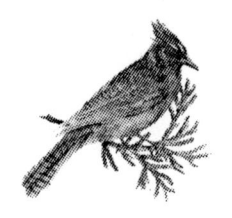

Day 3

Daddy's home!

"People say that what we're seeking is a meaning for life...I think that what we're seeking is an experience of...the rapture of being alive."
Joseph Campbell, *The Power of Myth*

Poppa has made his decision. Father and son are home and this woman's heart is whole again.

Then began the lessons of oxygen, cannulas and condensers, pain pills and the life of the dying in our family. We already knew that night time was when the pain attacked as Poppa sank into deep sleep and his heart seemed to labor the more.

All day I kept hearing my voice, as a little girl, chirping: Daddy's home! Daddy's home!

Buddy-dog would not leave Poppa's side, laying his head on his lap, nudging and licking his hand when it became still, listening to every word Poppa spoke, every breath he took, every snore he made.

Such a picture of devotion. Buddy-dog has taught me much about starting each day with a brand new heart and about always being ready to love, bottomlessly.

*   *   *   *   *

When the alarm chimes in our bedroom, we rise and turn on our light so Poppa knows we are awake. We don our slippers and robes and stumble together over to his cabin to calm Buddy-dog and administer to Poppa's needs. Then we plod back to sack out until the next time.

Now the thoughts of our own mortality linger just below the surface; when we examine our own wills and last testaments; when we exchange ideas of how we'd like our remains disposed and what sort of celebrations we'd like to sponsor.

With all the changes in our routines we have been wall-to-wall busy. One time, when we were in Poppa's cabin, in the middle of a visit from neighbor Evelyn Person (who shared the same birth date with Poppa), he woke up suddenly and growled: "What does a feller have to do to get fed around here?" We all chuckled, and Evelyn chatted with him while we prepared a light meal.

Poppa has been quite chipper until the pain attacks. With the new medications VMH prescribed, his appetite had returned and he has managed to crack a joke or two and even smiled at ours. He has been able to rise from his bed, walk about his cabin and out to his porch for fresh air. He has been as coherent as before, and while his faculty for understanding context and continuity in the here and now has waned noticeably, he still spins those marvelous memories.

David has had to suffer through infuriating bouts of frustration and helplessness as bureaucrats deny a nutrient-rich beverage because the doctor hadn't written the right percentage of food intake, or refuse a wedge pillow because the patient hadn't met the percentage of invalidness.

The daily Logs and my Journal

Ever since Poppa's knee replacements, David and I had kept a detailed log of Poppa's state of health and all the medications we'd given him, noting when given and what reactions, if any, he had to them. Having that legal pad on the shelf next to the bottles and weekly pill boxes for his morning, afternoon and evening doses, helped us keep track of what we were doing, and not have to rely on our memories which, at times of long watches, were faulty.

These logs were extremely useful when calculating David's working hours for the DSHS agency who paid him a minium wage for being this Senior Citizen's care giver. It was also vital when talking with Poppa's doctor, and later, the home health nursing team.

I have ever been a journal-keeper since I was given my first diary, complete with pencil and key, for my sixth birthday. I would check with the logs as I recorded how I felt each day and what it all meant to me.

The Log excerpts signify how time began to stand still, as each day expanded from the necessary busy-ness of being in service, to a broader experience of being in the present, of my becoming more conscious of living in the moment, of each breath we took.

Poppa's chores

We had always encouraged Poppa to do some chores each morning when he awoke, and most days he was glad for something to do.

The first thing Poppa would do on rising, was always to use one of the three urinals set in a bucket beside his bed. Then he would find his slippers tucked neatly beneath his bed, and walk across his cabin to open his front door to greet the new morning, and let Buddy-dog out for his first sniff of the day.

As Poppa made his first foray of the day, he would punch the coffee maker's button in passing. He often commented on how much he enjoyed the smell of coffee of a morning.

If Poppa was feeling chipper, he would carry the bucket of urinals into his bathroom and empty his overnight waters into the toilet. Then he would make his way to his recliner to take his dose of prunes and start on his first pint of water with his first set of pills. Many of Poppa's pills had to be taken with food and the prunes seemed a natural way of doing that. Besides, Poppa was mighty partial to prunes. If he had his way, and sometimes he did, he would eat prunes all the day long!

When Buddy-dog was done with his morning's sentry sniffs and markings, Poppa would get up and let him in, and replenish his bowl from the food bucket. If it was raining, Poppa had a special towel with which he'd dry off his companion. They made a fine game of it. I often would hear Poppa's chuckle at Buddy-dog's antics.

Then it was time to dress. For years, Poppa would methodically clothe himself in a ritual for which I could not stand still. Usually I timed my own chores to arrive when he got to his socks and shoes. Some mornings, I helped him with those and then had him lie back on his bed to do his leg exercises. Only in the last year of Poppa's life did I find him, more mornings than not, only halfway through the job by the time I came over after putting feed out for the critters.

On the days Poppa was full of energy, he'd clamber on board his ancient exercise bicycle, which we had permanently screwed down to the floor, and which he used as a clothes horse at night, as well as a prop to balance himself when he got out of bed. Poppa had named the old thing Charlie, and would pedal away for about half an hour, chatting with Buddy-dog and looking out of the window at the critters feeding.

Daddy's home!

David's e-mail to family and friends

> Hi All,
>
> I'm back from five days in Seattle at Virginia Mason where the doctors have declared that Poppa is terminal. Glad to be home in our cabins in the woods with the rain pouring down and the darkness of the early evenings.
>
> Poppa is resting, well attended by all sorts of machines, tubes and stuff, recovering from the 6 hour drive. Rebecca got a smile out of him today and he's eating a little more each day. The "heartburn" is, of course, angina and we now have appropriate medications to deal with the pain.
>
> I am very tired from loss of sleep and jumping through all the hoops of making the necessary arrangements that are going to be needed.
>
> I will try to keep you all posted as things develop and I have time. LoveanlateryaBro

Log excerpt for Day Five of The Watch

Sunday, October 31

07:00am "Good morning, Sweetheart!" Bright eyed and bushy tailed. Wanted a rubbing alcohol bath. Drank thirstily: 250cc water and 240ccD coffee. 400cc urine

08:30 Served him his favorite breakfast: ate it all plus all the milk!

09:35 Gave him his morning meds w/100cc water. 250cc urine

Noon Lunch w/Rx beverage.

02:00 Back to bed, willingly drank 250cc chilled water. Dozing.

04:03 Pain. 1 nitro tab.

04:10 5% reduced. 2nd nitro ab.

04:20 30% reduced.

04:24 Pain "...pretty near gone."

05:20 Meds with Rx beverage. Wants no food.

08:30pm Gave him his final meds of the day. No pain. Ready for bed.

Slept through night & so did we!

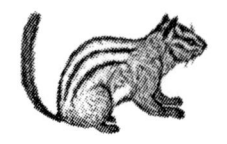

Day 5

Good morning, Sweetheart!

When I first met Poppa for that early breakfast at Gwennie's, he had greeted me with: "Good morning, Sweetheart!" And eagerly offered up his old man's cheek for my kiss. Unless he was feeling low or had had a bad night, this was how this Old Soul greeted me every morning.

Now, all those books that have been catching my eye on our library's shelves, begin to make sense, although no book I had yet found, told me nearly as much as the team of home health nurses in attendance.

At all hours of the day or night, in everyday words, these kind and conscious nurses, whom we came to consider as our sisters and brothers (yes, there are male nurses these days!) listened to our worries; offered solutions; asked clear questions; chuckled at our descriptions and efforts to lighten our mood; patted our shoulders, and told us how well we're doing. I really do mean conscious, for these folks were not only conscientious, they were fully aware of both what life and death in the here and now meant, and what we novices were feeling as we three navigated toward this death.

Today, I walked over to Poppa's looking forward to his gravelly-voiced welcome. As I lingered on his porch, listening to his snores through the door, I suddenly remembered Mrs. Fish, and a huge wave of fondness and laughter filled me, for she had put me through my paces!

Mrs. Fish had lived across the lane from the doctor's practice in Port Townsend, where I worked as its office manager and managing editor for *The Townsend Letter for Doctors*, a magazine we published ten times a year. For years she and I had waved at each other as we got out of our cars or put the garbage out. Occasionally, as I'd get out of my Pinto, she was carrying in groceries. If my arms were free, I'd dash over and help with her bags. Over those years I'd also noticed that no one ever came to visit this neighbor.

One summer morning, as I was coming to work, I heard a sharp, old lady voice calling. Mrs. Fish was leaning out of her Dutch door, beckoning to me.

As I arrived at her door, I got a whiff of something strong, and when she drew me in, the odors that blasted my nose took my breath away. Urine, burnt grease, cat litter and something else. Having run my own professional home cleaning business in California before moving up to the Northwest, I had a keen nose for household smells. Before I got the job with the doctor, I continued administering my magic in people's homes with the skills my mother and her sisters had taught me. After I graduated high school, I won a two-year scholarship to an art school, which worried my mother so much that she sent me off for a year to her sisters' families in Portugal. Upon my return to sooty old London, I had fallen into a deep depression, and my mother had sent me to secretarial college; admonishing me to "...earn your keep and keep out of trouble...you'll always be able to fall back on that." And I did, when I interviewed for the doctor's job and dusted off that other set of skills.

Chattering all the while about her trials and tribulations, Mrs. Fish showed me her bedroom where she'd had an accident and hadn't made it to the bathroom in time and, "...like a dog with the runs," she had squirted all over her bed and carpeting, leaving a trail across the dining room to the bathroom.

I was stunned and simply stood there surveying the mess, wondering where to start. In answer to her repeated appeals, I told her I'd be back, that I had to go get some things and I bolted out of that stagnant home, and sprinted back to the clean and comfortable doctor's practice. The good doctor was in between patients, preparing a snack in the kitchen, as I burst back in. We devised a plan of action.

"If you need me, I'll come on over." He had said, munching on a sandwich.

I gathered up a box of latex gloves, rolls of paper towels, plastic bags and aprons and, as I headed back to Mrs. Fish's home, I planned how to be in service to this elder's needs.

My first mistake was to assume Mrs. Fish had hot running water. Yes, she had a 50-gallon water tank, and yes, she had all the electricity she needed, however, she'd been in the habit of turning off her water heater until bath day.

Mrs. Fish would have to get used to the idea that every day from now on, was going to be a bath day.

Waiting for the water heater to do its thing, I swabbed down the cruddy tub and found her linen closet, setting out fresh towels after inspecting the ones already hanging on the racks and relegating them to the hamper.

Mrs. Fish fussed behind me, wafting her particular aroma right under my nose, all the while muttering about how hard it was these days to get good help. Once, I almost unbent from my task to stare her in the face and give her what-for. I decided to direct that surge of anger toward her filthy toilet.

Mrs. Fish had had the smarts to lay one of the 20 years of newspapers stacked about her dining room, on the seat she occupied while eating or watching television. As I swept past, I folded up the soiled paper, stuffing it into a garbage bag and laid down a fresher edition from a few years earlier. Then I approached her dank and dim bedroom again. I laid down more newspapers on her watery trail and tore her bed apart, stuffing her cold water washer with the soiled linens, adding a liberal dose of soap and bleach.

That was my next mistake. I was to find out that bleach and urine do not make for a kind blend on old, paper-thin flesh, and when Mrs. Fish developed what I could only call a diaper rash, or galling, out came the cornstarch, and I ceased adding bleach to her intimate wear.

With her whines accompanying me, I made Mrs. Fish show me where she kept her sheets and pillow slips. Remaking her bed was a lesson in humility and history. She had a particular way she liked her sheets tucked in, she didn't believe in those newfangled fitted things; each pillow had to be fluffed and laid just so before the top sheet could be placed. When it came to her ratty collection of blankets, reeking from the ages, her particularity reached a climax. I couldn't have cared less about what she wanted to sleep under. Luckily, by then, the water heater had completed its cycle, and I could now march the weary old woman into her ablution center to dunk her sore, smelly old bones in some warm, clean water.

Mrs. Fish did not like bathing, not at all! "Waste of good water!" I couldn't help laughing as I bundled up her soiled socks and housecoat, and prepared to help her into the huge old, claw-footed tub.

What a tiny little body! In my prime forties, I could only wonder at the determination and life brimming from this gaunt and ancient vessel. Would I be so alive when I was her age? Just how old was she, anyway? I said a blessing that she kept her hair short.

Mrs. Fish was fiercely modest and ordered me out of the room. So I started another load of laundry and cleaned up the cat droppings, tossed the litter into another bag and freshened it up. I had yet to see Mrs. Fish's furry friend. I swept up the scattered dry food that had tumbled out of the fallen bag, and turned to look at the kitchen.

That was my next mistake. In all my years of professional cleaning I had not come upon a kitchen in such a state. Decades of frying grease and nicotine created a patina of dull orange on ceiling, walls and cabinets. The electric range looked like it belonged in a museum and every counter top was covered with brittle, carefully placed paper towels. Across the floor were the trails Mrs. Fish made from dining room to back door, from sink to range, and all around the bottom of the counters. Everywhere else on that floor was a sticky, sickly shade of grey.

By then Mrs. Fish was calling that she was done and ready to get out of the tub. That was when I saw her leg ulcer and the bruises. I made a note to call the doctor over here for a look-see.

Dried and dressed (I didn't say anything about her lank, unwashed hair that day), Mrs. Fish was hungry. What she wanted was her instant coffee with evaporated milk and sugar, spoonfuls of it! While she ordered me to prepare something to eat, she sat at the freshened dining room table (Oh, I'd given it a swipe in passing) and indulged in her first cigarette of the day.

What Mrs. Fish wanted to eat was a blast from my past. Heated baked beans with a can of little sausages dumped into it. She also wanted toast. She owned neither toaster nor microwave, simply a collection of huge, heavy cast iron pots and pans that you had to be Hercules to handle!

When I opened the bread bag, I discovered a lively colony of penicillin and was about to toss it when her sharp wit caught on, and she ordered me to dump it all in that baking dish over there, along with the rest of her scraps. That was for her birds. She didn't know what her birds would do without her.

Weeks later, as I was brewing a pot of my own real tea in the kitchen at work after a marathon night of laying out the magazine, I was to learn who her birds really were. Out she came in that daybreak, screeching like a banshee. In a sudden rush of silent shadows, a flock of seagulls arrived, hovering in the lane. In a ritual of many years training, they swooped and caught what she lobbed up at them. Pacific Ocean seagulls are huge and they jostled skillfully for Mrs. Fish's scraps. When all the scraps were thrown, the cacophony they set up was enough to wake the dead.

Every pot and pan in Mrs. Fish's kitchen was coated with culinary history, and the smoking reek when I heated up her frypan, gagged me. Apparently I had made a perfect meal, for she dove into it with relish. As she lit up her postprandial cigarette, I was to witness a ritual I'd not seen before. Out came her false teeth, which she cleaned by dunking into her glass of water, all the while dragging on her smoke with her toothless mouth. With much smacking of lips, she then wiggled her teeth back into place. *I would have to try that one!*

The sound of me washing up drew her into the kitchen, and she stood at my elbow admonishing and directing as to how she wanted it done. *Such a ritual!* I asked her why all her counters were covered with paper toweling. Her cat liked to walk everywhere, and that was her way of keeping her counters clean. I peeked under the paper. Sure enough, her counters were the cleanest surfaces around!

That first day, I stayed over six hours, picking up and cleaning, tidying and mopping. As with everything else, Mrs. Fish's mop was a study in ancient filthiness, and her janitor bucket, complete with ringer, had to be washed before I could use it. The linoleum in that kitchen must have arrived with the first settlers.

I called the doctor to come over, and he inspected her leg. She wouldn't let him see the bruises, although she relished his attention. She said they were from falling down when she got dizzy. He had brought over some supplies and taught me how to work on her ulcer. He then took her vitals and pronounced her in pretty good shape for the shape she was in.

Mrs. Fish was content.

He vanished after about half-an-hour, and I let Mrs. Fish know that I would have to be going soon.

By then it was afternoon and she was ready for teatime.

Teatime with Mrs. Fish was a time warp. My years among the English prepared me well for her ritual and in no time at all, we were ensconced in her sun room, with the afternoon light glowing through nicotine-coated windows, sitting on dusty, dainty pre-WWII art nouveau chairs with American knickknacks all about and a wall of shelves laden with African Violets in bloom, a curtain of greens, magentas, pinks and purples.

Teatime was when the cat appeared. A semi-feral, uncut marmalade male who sauntered in, and took over Mrs. Fish's entire attention until he'd gotten his dose of tea — heavy on the sugar and evaporated milk and the sardine sandwich Mrs. Fish had exhorted me to prepare. All the while she chain-smoked in that warm, bright room of bamboo, faded prints, scentless flowers and fascinating pottery: 1930s porcelain autos, dozens of salt and pepper shakers, fan vases out of which stuck flower cadavers, plates from Southern states, and clocks, none of which were keeping any kind of time.

Teatime, and the lady of the house was washed and fed. Surrounded by her mementoes and crooning to her cat, she was ready to reminisce. The story she told me that afternoon held me entranced.

She had been the apple of her Daddy's eye in a Mississippi port town. Her Daddy and his brothers had owned a merchant shipping line. When she was old enough she began to work in her Daddy's office.

When she recounted the first time she ever set eyes on Captain Fish, she glowed and her smile was beatific. Romance bloomed. Apparently they looked at each other and just *knew*. Daddy was not pleased, he had higher plans for his Little Girl. She was, however, adamant and her Daddy had to concede.

For their honeymoon, Captain and Mrs. Fish set sail on one of Daddy's ships, for a long, leisurely steam around the Pacific Ocean, delivering and picking up all sorts of cargo, with the intention of ending up in Japan, where they had booked a hotel suite, and were expecting to stay until the ship had taken on its return load.

Months later they steamed into harbor and were promptly interred, separately, in a Prisoner of War Camp. Newlywed Mrs. Fish was to spend the first years of her marriage incarcerated with other American and English women and their children. She could talk to her husband only through a wire fence for a few minutes once a day.

The carcass of her Daddy's ship was still there in 1945, and Captain Fish was ordered to bring it back. Husband and wife, along with hundreds of POWs and wounded soldiers, plus a military crew and nursing staff, steamed across the Pacific, through the Panama Canal and limped home to peace and a family reunion.

Mrs. Fish wouldn't talk about those years in the camp. She focused on their homecoming, on their life afterward, on their sorrow at not having any children, and their eventual retirement up here in the Pacific Northwest.

By then, the sun had gone behind the trees in her garden, and the room was cooling down. She wanted to move into the dining room for her evening of television. I helped her there, with a detour to the bathroom. When I turned on the TV, I noticed that the button and the aerial were broken. When the screen brightened, it was shrunken, distorted and the picture was a purple and green plaid. This TV was dying. I suggested she buy a new one, an idea that had not occurred to her.

That was when she directed me to her checkbook and I discovered this was one well-heeled little old lady. I was ordered to balance her book, she was getting mighty tired of that chore, and go, this very evening, to buy her a television. Oh, and by the way, see that shopping list, right there beside the checkbook? Why didn't I just pick those things up too? She'd even sign a check for me and call the store to OK my shopping for her.

That was my next mistake. Shopping for her without first getting all the details. Every single item on that list, and there were more than twenty, had to be exactly what she wanted. The brands, the sizes, the types and the quantities. She knew precisely what she wanted and resented substitutes. It didn't matter if the brand item cost more, she wanted that brand in that quantity; she wanted those types of paper towels and that kind of toilet paper; this brand of sardines; evaporated milk; baked beans; cocktail sausages; instant coffee; instant tea; sugar; bread; butter; cat food; cat litter, etc., etc.

I did do right by the television, though. She was entranced with its color, its size, the ease of turning on and off and its sound. She didn't bat an eye at the price.

Within a week, Mrs. Fish had me hooked. I was on the phone to every agency I could think of to give succor to this Senior Citizen and give me some relief. With two children in Junior High School, a job that was more than full time and a monthly publishing deadline, even I, in my Super Woman Decade, could not carry alone this fragile Old Soul.

Suddenly, out of the woodwork appeared all sorts of industrious bureaucrats. They dropped off daily meals at which Mrs. Fish scoffed, at first. They helped me start one almighty spring cleaning. Nurses showed up twice-weekly to care for the ulcer, which was healing just fine, and to wash and care for our aging charge.

Soon, I was able to visit in my regular work clothes rather than in my heavy-duty cleaning gear. Soon, the piles of newspapers holding up the walls and weighing down the chairs, were bundled and hauled away. Soon, new bedding, bathroom fixtures and cooking utensils filled her brightening home. In time windows were professionally cleaned. At first Mrs. Fish shrieked at the light that poured in. Curtains were cleaned and rehung. The chandelier over her dining table was lowered, washed and the coated dead light bulbs replaced. Mail was brought in and garbage taken out daily.

Mrs. Fish was rejuvenated with all her visitors, all the new things going on around her. She no longer had to struggle with her bank account; with cast iron pots and pans she could no longer lift; nor with the laundry which she could no longer remember to do.

Mrs. Fish presided over her slew of servants as if to the manner born. Autocratic and flirtatious she demanded, reprimanded and commanded our attention and our obeisance to her every particular whim.

In time, I bowed out, visiting weekly for a cuppa in her sunroom. She still smoked like a chimney—unfiltered Chesterfields. She still stirred four spoonfuls of sugar into her instant tea with evaporated milk, and still sipped that brew from 50 years old mugs brought from the galley of her Daddy's ship.

Beneath the grime reposed a shiny old coin. In the dining room I discovered a roll-top desk at which Mark Twain would have enjoyed writing. When I cleared off the dining table I found a Sears Roebuck classic, complete with Captain's chair and six ordinary unbroken seats. In the sitting room where Mrs. Fish no longer ventured, I unearthed china cabinets of assorted bric-a-brac older than Zeus. Beneath the newspapers, the table and the crud, I found carpets of such faded beauty and patterns as would grace a museum.

All in all, Mrs. Fish's home was once again a lovely place to live and, for a few more months, we enjoyed a companionship and working relationship that fed us both. Occasionally she would call me over for this emergency or that, usually around the uncomfortable struggle with her bowels and her lack of water intake. Mostly, it was that quiet time in her sun room, with her foul tasting tea and her strong flavored smokes, after a hard day of work and before I hurried home to my children, where she would regale me with her week's misadventures. Once in a while, something I'd say would rankle her and I'd catch that haughty look of deep offence, and she would emphatically change the subject.

Then one cold, spring day, when the sunroom was heated only by blasting air from her furnace, she became angry about something and gave me such an evil eye, I knew I wasn't coming back. I can't remember what it was about. Had it been something unforgivable I'd said? Had I overstepped my station in her life? Was it because she had finally met my children, when they had come to her back door one day after they had missed their school bus, and needed a ride home? Or was it her way of saying goodbye?

Whatever it was, she swept me out of her life, wouldn't let me wash up our dishes, hurried me out of her door. I let it be. I did keep up with the agencies, and I noticed when the nurses parked in the carport or when the Meals-On-Wheels came to deliver. I did watch for the cleaning girls and the deliveries of necessities from the local store.

One morning, late the next autumn, I noticed an ambulance and a police car quietly parked outside in the lane, no sirens, no lights. I saw a half dozen men and women, in various uniforms, milling to and fro as they wheeled a gurney into that kitchen door through which I'd passed so many times.

As I watched from the window of my office, I saw the body bag on the gurney. I saw the agency worker lock the back door from the outside, with Mrs. Fish's cat yowling in a travel cage at her feet. I watched as everyone drove away. And that evening, before I headed home, I noticed no lights came on in the house across the lane.

I looked for Mrs. Fish's obituary in our local newspaper, and learnt a few facts I hadn't known about this woman's long life. A month later I read about an auction of Mrs. Fish's worldly goods. I bid and paid for two of her galley mugs, and one of her African Violets.

* * * * *

Now, I stood Watch with my beloved as his father slowly made his way out of this world, with a grace and gentleness that brought tears to my eyes. Mrs. Fish had died one night, quite alone, and her passing went unremarked by neighbors. The differences with Poppa's dying made me wonder about how we live our lives, in what emotional climates we choose to abide, from which platform we decide to make our exit.

As an Adoptee, Immigrant and a Registered Alien for many years, the idea appeals to me that we all come into this life as immigrants, aliens to the mysteries of Life on Earth and our job is to adopt civilization and learn how to be the best humans we can; to transform ourselves from naked aliens into accomplished people, to be the best at who and what we are before we get our ticket to ride and head out on the next leg of The Grand Adventure.

I think some of us have decided to be the best nags, drunks and ne'er-do-wells we can imagine. Just as some of us feel called to be the best parent, soldier, spouse or millionaire. Some choose being best at a lot of things; some at a few. Whatever we choose, wherever we travel, we live to the fullest, although I have seen folks so shut down, and a-tremble in their nests, that they've become the best examples of scaredy-cats! What stories we all will take home to Mother Spider!

Sometimes, as I tended to this frail old feller, (a feller, out here in the Northwest forests, is a tree faller, otherwise known as a lumberjack. It was one of Poppa's many skills) I had the image of him with his ticket in his huge gnarled hand, sleepily biding his time in the Waiting Room at the Cosmic Station, until his number is called. David and I were his flight attendants, there to serve him snacks, ease his bodily needs, crack a few jokes and tell him he was loved in this lifetime.

While in service at this home death, I would feed the Steller's Blue Jays and the Townsend Chipmunks on the picnic table in front of his window, and throw ball for his Buddy-dog, so Poppa could watch his beloved companion leap and catch it on the fly, and bound on back to me to give it, as he was taught, everso gently into my hand.

Log excerpt for Day Six of The Watch

Monday, November 01

06:46am "Good morning, Sweetheart!" Poppa wide awake. Washed him down. He was able to take care of his privates. Asked for an alcohol rub especially on his back. Settled again he refused water, asked for a cup of coffee. Night bag 1200 cc yellowish. I left him in peace & went to set feed out for the critters on the table outside his window.

07:30 Moved him to his recliner. Gobbled up prunes & Rx drink.

08:20 He dug into his breakfast of grits & eggs, slurped down another cup of coffee (4 ounces only this time).

10:00 AM meds 250cc H20. Out: 350 cc yellow/moderate smell.

Noon Home health nurse arrived to give us all flu shots. Poppa back on bed. BP 110/58. Took a blood draw. Says we're doing fine. Had more forms. Called the doc for a morphine Rx. The doc's nurse said the Rx was at Chinook Pharmacy.

01:15pm Rang alarm. Needs help to the toilet for a BM. 8" soft, pale, no smell. Able to wipe himself. At his chair he drank 250cc water. Ate half a sandwich & half an apple+Rx drink. Slept.

04:00 Took favorite dinner: small salad, hamburger, pickle & 4 ounces of canned fruit salad. Ate it all up! No vomiting!!

07:00 Last Rx beverage of the day. Wanted to stay up & watch a program about the history of combine-harvesters.

08:00 Bedtime. Let Buddy-dog out. David changed condom catheter, connected nighttime bag. Alcohol rub on back & heels. Changed pjs. Washed daytime supplies. Tidied up.

09:00 Night Rxs. Tired of drinking. Said his feet were cold so we rubbed them. Ankles swollen, put on socks, raised the bed foot. Let in Buddy-dog. Kissed Poppa good night.

11:00pm Check up: sleeping, snoring.

A surprisingly pain-free day!

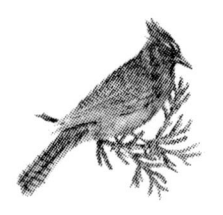

Day 6

The Certificate of Impending Death

Poppa was sometimes quite unable to give us any answers when we asked him how he was doing. More often than not, he would murmur, "I know, Son, I just don't know." It sounded as if it was hard for him to focus, and even harder for him to find the words to explain or describe how he was feeling. We rapidly learnt to read what his body had to say, even if his mind and mouth couldn't tell us.

It astonished me, when great swells of affection would roll through me like gusts of wind. I would be washing his feet, emptying his urine bag or combing his hair, and I would look upon his wise old face, his extraordinary hands, and simply want to hug and hold him as I had done with my babies. "There, there, Poppa. All is well. It's just your body that's dying, your spirit is getting ready for its next adventure."

Tending Poppa at this time, reminded me of the last weeks of gestation, when all I wanted to do was get away from the hectic world with its insistent noise, and pay undivided attention to what my body was going through.

Sometimes, however, I thought of all these years I'd tended to Poppa's needs as he became less and less of this world, and the resentment that surfaced, shocked me. Was it just because he was a man and expected women to take care of him? Was it just because he was a man of his generation and didn't know any better? Was it just because he was an Elder who had earned such succor?

As I had tended my daughter and son in their growth from infants to toddlers to children to teenagers, I had spurts of that same resentment: "Start taking care of your life. I'm not your servant, I'm your mother!"

Poppa had ever been polite to me, asking instead of ordering. Thanking instead of ignoring, and I often wondered how the father of my childhood would have been. I wondered if, at fifteen, I could have, should have been allowed to help in this way, and faintly would come the memory of the tears I had shed for my exile from that sacred time in my family, when our father's remains were being cared for.

Now, the Cosmos had decided I was old enough, and I stepped beside my husband as he tended the death of his father. I listened to David rant and rave against bureaucracies that had him jumping through petty hoops, as if there was all the time in the world.

I'd listen to this son wonder at becoming his father's father, taking care of his every need from money to doctors, from food to clothes and such intimate details as bowel movements, washing his penis and foreskin, putting on and taking off the condom catheters, helping him brush his teeth or shave. And, as I realized I had become my husband's father's mother, I remembered the vow I had made when we married; not just the ones between us as a couple, for that vow had included caring for my husband's father for the rest of his days. Do we ever really, really know what we promise to do? Easy words encompassing difficult actions: until death do us part.

Today, a new member of the home health nursing team gave us more instructions on condom cathetering, and more information on the medications amassed on the shelf like a pharmacy. She told us to also start logging in Poppa's output of urine, which we were now to sniff for aroma and gauge its color, as it would be changing in quantity, color and smell as his body's systems began to shut down.

Poppa engaged the nurse in gentle jokes as she went about checking his vital signs. Later, as she talked with us while Poppa dozed in his easy chair, the poltergeist bed started its growling comedy. Poppa woke up and we all watched in silence as the bed raised and lowered itself. Poppa quipped, with a broad grin, "Sure got a mind of its own, don't it!"

We were still fighting the red tape for a nutrient-rich drink which he loved. It was a pleasure to watch him slurp it all down. He just didn't seem interested in food, which was a major signal, one which the nurse assured us was quite normal.

With Poppa's vitals logged in, he was settled in his fresh bed with a snack on his lap table. The alarm button was taped to the guard rail within easy reach, so we retired to our cabin where the nurse made calls for more equipment. For the other things, we would have to drive to Port Angeles, and borrow from the Hospice warehouse as no prescription could be written for them.

Then we listened as the nurse proceeded to worry the socks off of us by asking what our plans were. Naturally, we thought she meant what we were going to do for the next few months.

"No, no. I mean for the next week or so!"

"Why?"

"Because Lincoln doesn't have months." David and I looked at each other. I felt as if a huge hole had opened up in me. I reached for my husband's hand.

"Not that long?" One of us asked.

"I don't mean to scare you," she spoke gently, "but I've been studying his chart and his progress and, well, his spirit and I, well, don't see this going on for months. What are your plans?"

"Plans? For what?" My fix-it husband asked.

"His remains." That was when I realized the future was upon us. Suddenly, this life we had known and loved was about to change, not in some vague future—*now*! *This was it!* We were going to have to get used to the idea of Poppa dying quicker than we'd been told.

David's hand held mine tightly.

"I'll register the Certificate of Impending Death at the Court House tomorrow," the nurse assured us.

"Why?"

"That allows you to call the funeral home rather than the police."

"Why would we call the police?"

"Because it's the law in this state. When someone dies, and a Certificate of Impending Death has not been registered, the police must investigate and the body is taken away by ambulance for an autopsy. You'll be questioned a lot, maybe taken to jail. You don't need that!" She was emphatic as she dialed Poppa's doctor and, unlike when we called, got straight through to him. Apparently he was quite willing to sign the certificate.

"The next nurse will bring out your copy which you must display at all times on Lincoln's cabin door. You realize don't you, there's no calling 911 anymore? That your doctor isn't going to come out here? They don't do that anymore, you know."

It was a strange thought that the doctor would have seen Poppa each and every day, maybe even twice a day, had we put him in a nursing home or the hospital's long-term care ward. Because we chose to care for him at home, as he wanted, no doctor would be in attendance. "*Just as well!*" A little voice hissed in my head.

The interview proceeded, and the nurse eventually left, leaving scads of forms, pamphlets and telephone numbers. As she put her car in gear she leaned out of her window, "Remember, you can call our number anytime, day or night. There's always a nurse on duty to talk you through anything. Anything!"

* * * * *

Sometime in the afternoon, when we were in Poppa's cabin taking care of chores, what the nurse told us registered. We stood at the foot of his bed so he could see both of us at the same time, and David broached the subject.

"Poppa, it's all right. There're no bad feelings between you and me. You know I love you and I'll take care of you until you die and afterwards. We'll be just fine. You can go anytime you want. You've taken real good care of us. You know all your work is done. Now you can go home to your Lord. We'll be fine."

Poppa sighed, his eyes gleamed, tears oozed and almost a smile was on his lips. As I dabbed away his tears, I saw the relief of this Old Soul as his son gave him permission to die, about him saying it aloud and not running away, not mumbling it in a hurried moment.

Soon Poppa was dozing again, and a glow in the cabin grew that had nothing to do with the sunshine outside or the lights inside.

*   *   *   *   *

When I check on Poppa before I head for bed, I watch him sleeping and stroke his hand. Buddy-dog will want to go outside for another sniff and I'll set the heater's thermostat, check the oxygen machine and empty the urine bag. Then Buddy-dog will want in, and so I plod back home to our cabin.

David will be in his pjs, reading in his easy chair, sleepy with his medications. Now he'll be on duty. We snuggle for a bit. He'll doze and read the night away and then around 4am he'll come to bed, and I'll be up to take the morning shift.

Tucked into our bed, I say my prayers and wonder how I will feel when I've been told I'm going to die soon.

It's been a good day to be alive.

Snail-mail to Lincoln's far-flung relatives

Dear Family,

Lincoln is receiving calls on his new, hearing-impaired modified telephone, usually between 10–11am and 1–2pm local time. He's already received calls from his children in Alaska and was able to connect for a short while, the lower and the slower you speak, the better. He's receiving cards from folks wishing him well. We can print out any e-mail messages you send and he puts on his eyeglasses and reads them all, often!

Lincoln was up and about today, pain free. When you think about a charlie horse in your calf: imagine how grim and scary it must be to have that happen in your heart! His medications are taking effect, he's calmer and clearer, joking and remembering things. He had a great dump after a four day hiatus. You know, getting rid of that shitty city!

We've had some wonderful moments, when tears of gratitude and love have choked us all, lots of stroking and holding hands. He's even looking at us in the face again, no longer hidden away behind the pain and fear.

The farce with the hospital bed continues, although it seems to have formed an attachment to Poppa, and has become quite biddable! David's even figured out all the combinations of the buttons.

Lunch seems to be Lincoln's most hungry time. He's enjoying his booster beverage three times a day, reminds him of malts and he sucks them up through a straw, gleefully making lots of noise. Sometimes I catch him watching me to see if I'm annoyed. I grin because it's music to my ears, means he's finished it!

With loving thanks,

David & Rebecca & Lincoln & Buddy-dog too!

The comfort of cyber friends

All during this home death, the connection with my friends via e-mails was vital. Those words would glow from my monitor, offering comfort, wisdom and support. These friends could not take the time to drive out here. There would have been nowhere for them to stay anyway, and in the intensity of our hour-by-hour Standing The Watch, we could not have been so connected as when we wrote back and forth.

Deborah and I met a score of years ago when she was deeply wounded by the death of her oldest son in a car crash. I began cleaning her home and helping her heal. She and her husband often would come out to the West End for surfboarding and camping out, and they always stopped by for a visit.

Jane is a quilting bee friend from my Port Townsend years, who roams the wilderness with her photographer husband, and has kept our friendship alive with her emails.

Artie Carter made contact with David at a computer glitch deciphering chat room. They resolved many a problem as their friendship blossomed.

May had grown up along the road and had, one summer, brought her husband and children out to visit the house of her childhood nearby. On the urging of her mother and father, who had known David when he had first lived along the road, May had looked us, and became a cyber friend when she returned home. May was still recovering from Standing The Watch of her own father's dying, and pacing us through the Valley of Death, helped her heal from her own experience.

RR and I met during my women's spiritual movement years. Together we built sweat lodges, created ceremonies, and danced and drummed the nights away at the annual Long Dances high in the Olympic Mountains. When she feels the need for a quick vacation, she drives out to wander the beaches and forest, stopping by us for a visit.

Faina from Alaska, was a friend from my Port Townsend years. Our children had been in school together, and then she moved away to be near her grandchildren.

Donna is a friend of a friend, who likes to read and who simply stayed with me through The Watch.

Lynn came into my life when I interviewed her as part of my work for our website. The books she has written have changed my life. She consistently encouraged and mentored me during the writing of this book.

Carolyn also came into my life through our website, and has become my dear friend and touchstone.

*   *   *   *   *

My very dear May,

Wonderful, wonderful e-mail from you. It really helps that you've been there, done that! Yes, if you would send that Hospice leaflet, we'd greatly appreciate it. I'm getting books out of the library because right now I need to read things plain and simple. Hospice cannot help us, as we're too far out in the wilderness.

That sanity you wrote about is very real. Sometimes we find ourselves giggling and cutting up something weird, and in the next moment we'll have catches in our throats, tears in our eyes and lumps in our chests. It's all so exciting and adrenaline-rushing and sort of hurry-up and go nowhere.

We're both without appetite, although Poppa's eating well, when he's eating. He doesn't seem to be hungry later in the day. Breakfast is small, lunch is good and supper is a couple of bites. He's getting a nutrition-rich drink, which he loves. He's kept his sense of humor unless the pain comes. We've finally gotten the proper meds and he can be almost pain free now.

The worst thing now is coping with taking care of his remains in the manner he wishes! Whoever said life was dignified hasn't had babies or elders! Still, it's all a part of the rites, ceremonies and spirituality of living a conscious and content life.

We thank you so much for staying connected with us. That you speak so clearly to our needs is simply because you truly know. Interestingly enough, those who haven't yet walked through the Valley of Death with a loved-one, have only given me a line or two of their news or have been unable to respond at all.

Poppa's got his ticket for the next migration, the next step in the Wheel of Life or, as is closer to his philosophy, going home to the Lord. Now he's waiting for his flight to be called and we're simply earthbound flight attendants serving him coffee, tea and some comedy.

Take care and thank you for being there.
Rebecca & David & Poppa & Buddy-dog too!

E-mails of the day

Rebecca and Dave,

I am so sorry for Poppa, it is so hard to watch someone so astounding and sturdy suddenly get weak and feeble.

Our prayers are with you all, please keep us informed of his progress. With this letter know how much we are linked with you in this endeavor and may you always know how much we care. Mom and May.

* * * * *

Dear You'all,

Poppa is in our prayers, and I feel honored that you include me in your most trying moments. You paint a vivid picture that makes it easy to understand the feelings you are having, howling dogs and coyotes in tune with the siren and the cool moonlit air, with a desperate feeling of losing something you have held close for a very long time and aren't sure how you will proceed without. About a fist sized mass in your chest tightens up as if the heart is drawing up into one tight knot. May our Heavenly Father comfort you with the knowledge He's there with you, if for no other reason that I asked Him to be there for you and David (He answers prayers like that). May His arms encompass you and comfort you with His eternal love and His guidance is there for the asking.

Love and Peace be with you always, Artie.

* * * * *

Dearest Rebecca,

Every day I read and reread your letters and just wanted to let you know that I am reaching out to all of you through the airwaves during these painful days.

From what you write I wish that I could meet Poppa. He must be one fine man. I'm sure that you will be richer for having chosen the most difficult road.

Blessings on you. Donna.

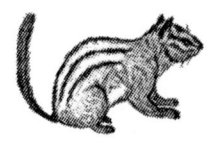

Our Gift

They don't make house calls

During a phone call with Poppa's sister-in-law in Missouri, the subject came up about doctors not making house calls the way Betty and I remember, even though we're thirty years apart in age.

In this streamlined age of HMOs and Medicare/Aid, we've sacrificed the comfort of the human touch for the long distance of red tape. Have we allowed our sense of community to erode by abdicating to the highest (or lowest) dollar rather than maintaining our right to have rites?

After this wise woman murmured, "They don't do things like they used to...things sure have changed." I ventured that Poppa's pastor also didn't make house calls. There was a long silence over the line, and I could hear this dear lady, whom I've never met, sigh and gather up her resolve to give me comfort. I wasn't raised in Poppa's traditions and I don't know the prayers for his soul's ease.

Another sign that tells me we're in trouble as a society has come to my notice while Standing This Watch and is ironic, if far more saddening.

As we live over a two-hour drive along winding wild roads, from the understaffed Port Angeles Hospice team, we were beyond its reach, and the nearer branch in Forks had just closed down. We had been directed, however, to call the Forks caregivers whenever we needed ease in our stress. We were assured they would speak with us. At one particularly crucial phase of getting the arrangements sorted out, I made that call.

When you are tending the dying, the essence of time is counted in minute increments; days of a week dissolve, as do the hours to a day. Thus, I was unaware I was calling on a Sunday. I shared some of our concerns with the ex-hospice worker, asking her for insights. She was oddly noncommital until suddenly, she interrupted to say that her ride to church was there, and she had to go. Before she hung up, she brightly chirped: "Call me anytime you're worried!"

I was, in an earlier incarnation as an office worker, ruled by the clock. Raising kids through the school system is also a study in abiding to an artificial schedule. At this hour thou shalt be here doing this; after this time, your life is your own.

One of the reasons I love sitting in old churches is their sense of timelessness. For hundreds of years, according to the way humans count time, these houses of worship have stood waiting. Enter their doors, find a pew, set your world-weary body down, and time will dissolve.

Being in the presence of the dying feels much the same.

The other ironic moment was when we called an out-of-state relative to let her know Poppa was fading fast. She answered in hushed tones, advising us she was entertaining the women elders of her church, and would call us back when she had time.

My beloved and I were learning that the very definition of dying is that you no longer have any time. Rather, time has you!

I would sit at my computer, weary and weepy, deeply in tune with the here and now of this home death of a beloved Old Soul who was born during a hot Midwestern summer thunder-and-lightning storm, on his parents' bed before the War to End All Wars, and I'd ponder on the irony that it is more important to ride to church than to speak with someone about the dying of their father.

I would sit at Poppa's side, deeply content wherein I found myself, and wonder at the kin who couldn't let members of her congregation know she'd be taking a once-in-a-lifetime call about the dying of one of the few left of his generation. "Ladies, my kin is dying and his son's on the line and needs to talk, I'll just be a few minutes." You'd think those church ladies would have understood.

Is this then the face of religion today? Long distance, buffered spirituality? Is this the real loss of community when the rite of dying at home is shunned? People dashing off to church instead of offering a dash of comfort? People handing out tea and biscuits instead of serving sympathy?

As I stroked this dear man's hand and gently laid my cheek upon it, I would murmur my love for him, and watch the panoply of emotions cascade across his wizening visage. See there, for a moment, the mischievous boy he once was before the seriousness of adulthood was thrust upon him. Now a momentary flicker of the young bully farmer, miner and logger, sure in the lay of his land. Still another moment rippled across this craggy face I'd learnt to love, and I'd clearly catch sight of the stern and devout missionary he was to become, once he had given his life to the Lord.

Now he murmured snippets out of parched lips which we soothed with ice chips: "...how's the beef here?" "...when are we going to build that fireplace, Del?" "...is Johnny here yet?"

Gone are the deadpan quips he would lob back at us: "How was dinner, Poppa?" "Good enough to make a young coyote sit up and sass his grandma!" "How are you feeling today?" "With all my fingers and toes!" "Can we get you anything?" "A nickel's worth of five dollar bills!"

* * * * *

What lessons this Old Soul has taught me in the few years I've known him. How relationships are grown, how love is nourished, and humor given. I've learned to wonder about time as I listened to Poppa's stories from before the First World War in the bread basket of America; when oil lamps were lit, water pumped by hand and babies born in their parents' beds. Of life before telephones, airplanes and televisions, not to mention computers, sliced bread and year-round vegetables. About listening to another's stories, just the way they're spoken, hearing their cadences, accents, and their own particular dialects and idioms.

I have also learnt how enduring I can be. Morning after morning after morning of emptying the night waters; cleansing an aging body; listening to biblical references and faint comedy that, had I not caught the twinkle in his eyes, I might have missed.

I have learned how to assure a beloved elder that what I do for him I have done for my children, and it is all part of loving life and loving him. Wiping up vomit or runny feces; cleaning soiled bedding and pjs, all of it is simply the process of life and has no meaning. Does that mean I like doing it? That my gorge doesn't spasm? Not at all. It simply means that it is my way of honoring this elder and making his final days and nights as loved and as comfortable as I can.

What I have learnt from this home death that I could not have learnt any other way, is that money and possessions aside, time is all we own.

That each breath is not to be taken for granted, rather it is to be relished with wonder.

That each blooming flower is an opportunity, and each falling leaf a memory.

That being present in our lives is enchanting. That as a human being in this Turn of the Wheel, there are thoughts and emotions that can darken the day or lighten the way, and I can do what I choose with those thoughts and emotions.

I have learnt that this home death is unusual rather than the norm. That the peace and light in Poppa's cabin as he ends his days draws me, and now that I am in concert with this time there is nowhere I'd rather be.

That the dying away of a body is part of being alive, and that soon enough it will be my turn.

That fear is a lively sensation which I can choose to feed, starve or use.

That simple gestures of affection: a hug, a kiss, a caress, are gifts to be daily given to our elders, just as we give to them our children.

That courtesy, in the face of death, is powerful.

That honoring one's promises is both testing and rewarding.

That my ability to love has nothing to do with anyone else, for to feel love I must first want to love and that is one thing I know, I want to live in love.

That evil is in the mind of the thinker, and can be held at bay by humor, and the courage to live kindly.

That I can think petty thoughts, and let them slide out of my mind, being neither moved to do anything about them nor encouraging them to linger.

That I can be generous beyond my imaginings with the only thing I truly own, my time, and that giving of my time to a loved-one who is dying, is really the only gift I have to offer.

That I yearn to live in the sacred, and that I am content to be a part of the Great Mystery, without using up my precious time defining It, naming It, for soon enough I will be It.

That I am much stronger than ever I thought I was.

* * * * *

Now, was the time for us in our marriage to offer all the comfort we could to each other. To tell each other our wishes for when we will be in the same place as Poppa—how we would like to die, our bag of bones disposed of and how we are remembered, celebrated. It was time to ponder together on The Great Mystery and say our prayers and sing our songs for a life well-lived. As was said in my English childhood—to celebrate "a good long innings," a reference to the mystical sport of Cricket that I so enjoyed as a youngster.

E-mails of the day

Hello you two,

Poppa is so blessed to have you and Dave by his side as he sleeps peacefully. Morphine has a lot to do with his throwing up, but it helps him sleep and rest comfortably.

I understand your weeping and weariness, you feel as though the only control that you have is over your emotions. Poppa's final job is to help you understand and to guide you through to understanding.

When his job is finished he will let you know. Take Care and get some fresh air, it will help. Love, May.

* * * * *

Dear Rebecca,

I wish there were something I could do to help you. This is very hard stuff.

We are holding space for all of you, I pray Lincoln will not be in too much pain and that he has a peaceful passing from this plane.

Love and prayers, Deborah.

* * * * *

OH Reb,

My heart goes out to you and David and Papa in these last days you spend together. I would love to have a short visit with you if life would allow...this is the sort of thing I do in my work these days...Hospice care...and I really love doing it.

I have been taught sooo much about the amazing capabilities of the human spirit. If you have any questions about his care or the nature of the dying process I promise to answer ASAP. I don't check my e-Mail on a regular basis but hubby is at it constantly and I can alert him to any messages received from you.

Is Papa in a lot of pain? If so, besides heart Rx he may need to have morphine &./or an Rx for anxiety. When I hear of night time pain in a dying person I think it has a component of fear to it.

Another thing I always tell my clients is that in this time they are in a powerful place between the worlds...between time and space...and that their main job is to finish up the business of this lifetime. In this powerful space they can go to any person, place or situation in their life and make amends, change things, whatever. In their drifting in and out of sleep/consciousness, I feel the dying person is accomplishing this work they need to do before the final crossover.

Also, the amount of fluid Papa ingests is one of the things that will tell you how close he is. Don't force food on him because as the body is shutting down it isn't of great importance and having to deal with the bowel function is often more trouble.

I hope things aren't going to be too much strain on you and David, make sure you take care of yourselves. It can go on for a while and be very stressful. I honor this journey of yours.

Love to you all...Hello to Papa from me...RR.

Log excerpt for Day Seven of The Watch

05:15am Poppa wide awake! No pain. 900cc fluid out, orange & strong smelling. Washed him & changed pjs. He wanted to get to his recliner for his coffee & breakfast. Drank all Rx beverage & ate a little. All stayed down, *praise be!*

10:00 Today Poppa refused to take his medications. I felt a huge shift in the cabin, as if a universe had just been let in; as if the sky had just opened. Tomorrow we'll have to tell the nurse when she gets here. Now I wonder what Poppa is thinking. For all his missionary years, has he any fears? *I don't dare ask.*

03:00 Not hungry for dinner, just some apple slices. A comfortable afternoon, dozed with Buddy-dog on his lap.

06:15 Time for bed. Decathetered. Showered. Recathetered. Fresh pjs. Rubbed his back. Cleaned up.

07:35 Chest pain. 1 nitro tab. No reduction+some water.

07:40 2nd nitro. Some reduction. *Isn't there a nitro patch?* Why is it so hard for doctors to get it about pain? The man's dying, who cares if he gets to like morphine more than is proper? Given the way this old man quaffs air, ain't no medicine around that'll stop his lungs before his heart gives out!

07:45 Pain gone. Hungry, wanted Rx beverage.

01:30 am Awake. Wanted nothing. No pain. We let Buddy-dog out for a sniff. Dry outside, coyotes calling. Talked some & kissed goodnight.

Each time we wonder if he'll be there the next time.

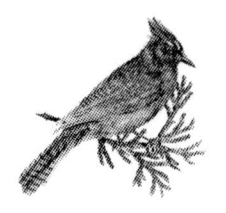

Day 7

Hear, O Lord, when I cry.

Psalm 27

Today, when we were both readying Poppa for his day, after settling him in his easy chair, he refused his medications.

David had stood there, with that little plastic cup in his hand into which he'd just poured the morning's dose of ten assorted pills, when his father looked up at him.

"Don't see the point, Son," Poppa muttered, stroking Buddy-dog's head which was lying in his lap on top of his quilt.

Outside his window, golden willow leaves were swirling like droplets of sun from the trees grown from our beloved friend Michael's cuttings. We'd kept the starts in a bucket of slurry until Poppa told us when and where to plant them. Beyond those now 20 feet high saplings was our cabin, from which we looked across into Poppa's to see how he was doing.

Two chipmunks scampered across the grass toward the picnic table for their breakfast. The blue jays were already there feasting.

Time stood still. Poppa had refused his medicines.

Here had come the final decision, the moment when Poppa made his last adult choice of his life, no more pills. No more swallowing those pebbles for his heart or digestion. No more for easing BMs or thinning blood. Not another horse pill of a supplement to keep his bones strong or his systems working. No more pills!

David and I looked into each other's eyes, leaned into each other for a moment. No more pills. Poppa had reached the end of his rope. He had punched his ticket and The Cosmic Conveyance was now in motion. *Gird up your loins, this was it! This was no test run, no dress rehearsal.*

I caressed Poppa's silver-white hair and kissed his grizzled cheek, nuzzling his scratchiness.

"Okay, Poppadum, no more pills. What would you like for breakfast?"

David turned back to the shelves we three had built from alders we had felled, sawn and planed. On the wall, beneath the counter light, hung an old, warped photograph of Poppa and David in a canoe on an Alaskan lake, taken when David was maybe twelve. I'd often seen Poppa staring at it.

Upon that shelf lay the note pad for the log we kept, and beside it was the pharmacopeia we'd amassed over the past months. David returned the pills to their day's slot, closed the lid with a snap and wrote in the log. Now Poppa was making it happen, and we would watch his body die.

* * * * *

Too tired all day to really think about it all. At times I think I'm just going through the motions and being there as present as can be. Sometimes I think it is the tiredness that has squeezed out, like wringing a wet cloth, all extraneous emotions, allowing me to come cleanly to Poppa's side; to tend him hour after hour bathed in the meditative glow of his final days. It feels as if we are cloistered away from the world, that we have stepped into a sacred haven where the lines between spirit and flesh have become blurred, softened and elastic.

When Poppa dozes, so do we. I'm glad there's no gardening or building projects, just wood and water to be brought in, and laundry to take to town.

*   *   *   *   *

My beloved is fond of saying: "You never learn something you're not going to use." When I married a man with an aging father, did I ever use what I had learned!

I used what I'd learnt from my double knee operations for when Poppa had his knee replacements. Back in the good old days of 1950s England, the orthopedic surgeons pronounced that I had "rugger" knees, meaning my injuries were most frequently seen in chaps who played Rugby. I had loved playing lacrosse, tennis, cricket and netball, until my knees began to dislocate at the slightest turn. The subsequent physical therapy had been Draconian and not designed for a girl. Armed with those memories and taking into account that Poppa was in his eighth decade of life, I designed a program which if relentless, was forgiving.

I used a lifetime of compensating for extreme myopia for when Poppa's vision rapidly began failing. Overnight, or so it seemed when I was six, I needed glasses. At the time the optician's reasoning for such a sudden loss of 20/20 vision was the bucketful of bricks that had fallen from my brothers' tree house upon my head. "Or," he had added, "It could have been the chicken pox, you had a very bad case of it."

I used what I'd learnt about compensating for hearing loss. In the same year, my mother had a stroke and became deaf in her left ear, and I had survived a diving accident in which I had landed on the water on my right side and burst the eardrum. I helped Poppa learn to listen and talk as his deafness increased, teaching him to lip read, and pay attention to what was being said. I was always amazed when he could hear us perfectly when some motor (perhaps the wood planer or the vacuum cleaner) was rumbling away, and which rendered me totally deaf. Yet, there he was, carrying on a normal conversation!

*****

Being in service to our Poppa's dying put me through my paces and then some! Everything I'd learnt from taking care of my family and then my children, came into use. Still, the only thing from my past which taught me about tending a home death, were the first few weeks of my children's lives, when the rest of the world faded away as I embraced motherhood with the fascination of the adopted, and the total attention I felt the celebration deserved. For this I had changed my entire life focus. I had quit my 9 to 5 job, bought into a secondhand book store where I sewed custom-made clothes and, apart from keeping the store open, my time was my own and thus I could attend to my newborn's needs.

Everything I learnt as a mother came into use for Poppa's needs, except it was all in reverse. From being able to take care of himself to being unable to do the simplest chores. Putting him at ease, letting him know, even as tears filled my eyes, that *that* is what family does; that I'd done it for my kids; no big deal, just the state of being human. Such dignity! Such sorrow!

Poppa was a man who loved to shave himself and slather on aftershave, so that the odor in his cabin would have us joking about it smelling like a cathouse! Here was a man who kept himself neat and tidy, and then had to allow another to care for his every need: "Lift your foot, Poppa." "Lean forward, dear." "Just a quick wipe and we'll be all done."

Being in service is why we hire professionals. It's not something we, ourselves, expect to do. Who then, do we expect to take care of our parents? Strangers? Is it easier to be a stranger taking care of another's intimate physical needs? If that were so, then why is mothering so vital to a child's wellbeing? Mothers are not strangers! Why then, when we are dying, should we be among strangers?

Being in service means performing all the life-support tasks and chores another person needs. Being in service requires deference, diplomacy and determination. It does not, however, treat us kindly for we must, more often than not, bear the brunt of folks unaccustomed to authority, who wield that scepter with scant decorum and little sense of team spirit. It takes a lot of practice to become a polite autocrat. Families' histories are full of stories of impolite, dictatorial and petty elders, as well as toddlers!

Being in service to Poppa's needs, sayings and proverbs, I didn't know I had learnt, echoed in my mind. Odd phrases from Shakespeare and the Bible, about the stages of man, about lank shanks and the nakedness of one's parents, would flitter through my mind. Thoughts would linger about honoring our elders, and about abandoning them when they need us the most.

Being in service isn't all dull, hard work! If your funny bone is developed, you can actually get someone to chuckle at the damndest moments. When the bowels play tricks before you can move, or the hand shakes too much to drink from a glass (that's why straws were invented) or the memory draws a blank when you most need it.

The ultimate goal of being in service is to be invisible, yet most of us prefer being seen for the work we do. I have no problem with being in service. My hackles rise, however, when I'm taken for a servant. I don't do servant well, no, not at all! I'm sullen and resentful and slow. Request of me, however, to do a service on behalf of the welfare of the family and you have a champion at your side!

Another predawn moment

Dearly Beloved Cyberspace Friends who are gathered around us at this time,

I'm on Watch now, my beloved at last come to bed to sleep. Poppa's also snoring soundly, his huge valiant heart pumping on, his old body jerking and quivering. His beautiful gnarled hands moving, searching for memories as his mind roams across nine decades.

I've turned off all the ringers on our phones and lowered the sound of the cordless one that I carry with me, this way whoever is sleeping can continue. My nerves are now so taut that I jump when that ringing begins.

This morning I wanted to run away. I wanted to take back that vow I'd made at our wedding. I wanted not to have to think of doses of medicines, of dangerous combinations.

Not to have to feel the anxiety about Poppa's pain or see the frown that tells me his heart is cramping.

Not to have to order Poppa to open his mouth, so I can give him some ice chips before he raises his tongue so I can drop a pill under it, nor watch out that in swallowing he doesn't choke or cough or dry heave.

Not wanting all this responsibility. This home deathing is hard work! *So, what else is new? Home birthing isn't a walk in the park either! You've done that, so grow up, girl! You asked for it, now get used to it!* Life isn't only a bowl of cherries, it's also a load of pits.

In time, my panic subsides. I know when I go into Poppa's cabin and do all of what worries me, I find it easier than I dread. Especially when I know doing these services, allows my beloved more precious minutes asleep to help heal his neuropathy.

Calls to and from relatives have been a study. One yackered on about how they'd just bought a new car and this and that, and could only afford so much for their share of the funeral arrangements. Another moaned about not being able to find an honest contractor to renovate her kitchen, and had just spent so much money she could only afford to send us a little. Another relative refused, in monosyllables, to engage at all, while another offered nothing. The only one to acknowledge what we're doing, and to offer half of the basic costs is himself, rather stretched.

So, my dear friends, keep connected, please. Your emails mean so much to us, another dawn and waking up to my first cup of tea.

E-mails of the day

Dear One,

I am so thankful to the universe for allowing me to cross paths with you. You are a light and inspiration to me and always have been. I wish there were something I could "do." I too will hold sacred space.

I don't sense you need help, but sharing as you said, which is wonderful and you said it so well, my dear. I know you all have the strength and wisdom to carry on, with spirit, through this difficult time.

Know though that we are here for you and if there is something that comes up that we can do, please let us know. I check e-Mail at least once a day.

Know that you have made a difference in this woman's life, also. And my man's, we both love you and hope to hear from you soon. Deborah.

* * * * *

Dear friend Deborah, I sense this is not a good time for company, we're very focused, quiet in our ways, in tune with this gentle moment. Keeping company with you this way is deeply wonderful, thank you for being there, you are a princess among women. I love you. xoxRxox

* * * * *

Dear Rebecca, Dave, Poppa, Buddy-dog,

I am so glad that you received some easement from my e-mail. I am sorry I can not take all the hurt away. It is very hard to go through each day wondering if it will be the last. Hang on to the giggling

and cutting up as you will need it, especially for Poppa. As the days wear on he will probably lose his sense of humor, and become a different person sometimes not even knowing who you are, especially if he is taking pain meds and the oxygen.

It is good that he is getting nutrition. Is he walking about or is he confined to the poltergeist bed? The pain meds and the drink will also cause his bowels not to move, but all of a sudden he will not be able to control them and the time then comes for Depends. My father was a very modest person but when it came to changing him I was the only one, outside of Mother, who he would allow himself to be seen by.

You're right in one instance, sometimes dying isn't dignified. Why do some elders have to go the whole course? I often asked myself, when Dad was in so much pain, is it for myself that I want to keep him going? Even when he was ready to go I wasn't, I hung on for him.

Make sure that you do get some fresh air in your lungs everyday and don't get over tired, if you find that the neighbors are willing to sit a spell with Poppa, let them, he will need the breath of air as much as you.

Everyone doesn't follow the same path so take what you need from the paper and leave the rest and don't borrow trouble.

Take Care and we are thinking of you.

Give Buddy-dog a hug he will need it also, he is sensing something. Mom and May

Log excerpt for Day Eight of The Watch

Wednesday, November 03
07:00am Wide awake & pain free, wonder of wonders! Enjoyed the bed bath & the alcohol rub down. Tickled the soles of his feet, today he jumped & chuckled. Perhaps all those medicines had numbed him out.

07:30 Managed an entire 250cc of water. Night fluid in the bag was 1800cc, dark yellow. Changed to daytime bag. Did clean-up ritual & helped him to his chair. Didn't want his prunes. That's a first, he surely loves his prunes!

08:00 Fiddled with breakfast: "...just not hungry." Drank all of his Rx beverage. Dozed.

11:30 Home health nurse arrived & Poppa was interested in meeting the new "feller." The nurse inspected our log, checked Poppa's feet, hands & eyes. BP 94/54 P60 irreg./Temp 97.4. Listened as we told him about Poppa refusing his meds. Nodded & said that was normal in people who were conscious & that the end would be soon.

01:00pm The loaner hospital bed delivered by Jim's Pharmacy. Poppa fiddled with lunch. Finished his Rx drink.

05:15 Wanted another Rx drink.

07:00 Ready for the night. Alcohol rub. Shoulders & heels red. Little in his catheter bag. Changed out catheter. Cleaned up.

A busy & mostly pain free day.

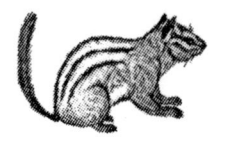

Day 8

With all my fingers and toes

Poppa spent the afternoon in his recliner watching his critters play and me planting bulbs. I purposely planted where Poppa could watch me. I didn't let him see me crying as I bent to Mother Earth, singing my Songs, placing those promises of life into her embrace. It was enough to comfort him, with his fading sight, simply to see a woman, bending down to earth, about her womanly work.

One of Poppa's favorite sayings, when he had been asked about how he was feeling, was to gruffly comment, "With all my fingers and toes!" One doctor was not amused and stared his old patient down, while another cracked a grin, patted Poppa on his back and cheered him on.

Well, this Old Soul hadn't been feeling much in the past year with his work-worn fingers, and both his hands shook so much sometimes he couldn't pick little things up. Fiddling with the television remote control had become a frustration. *How industry discounts our infirmities. Heck, even I have to peer and prod and poke the dam' things!*

Strangely enough, Poppa's feet were in fine shape. On the first Friday of each month, we used to drive him to the visiting podiatrist who cut and cleaned his toe nails, inspected for abrasions, blisters and numbness. The doc gave Poppa a good bill of health for his two old plodders. Now Poppa wore bed socks all the time. I'd change them out after I rubbed his heels with alcohol, and anoint his feet with lotion. Now he rarely responded when I tickled his soles.

For some reason I found anointing this Elder's feet an intensely sacred ritual. One that connected me with the host of women who have been there, done this. Images of the Christ doing the same would flash in my mind, reminding me of how such a simple gesture offers such deep comfort, respect, even loyalty. This was my husband's father, he whose wisdom has guided us in reclaiming this devastated triangle in the timber farms. His son, who had been a building contractor in another lifetime, encouraged his father to search his vast store of knowledge as we built our round cabins, the thinking and remembering as much for the wisdom as for exercising Poppa's stroke-damaged mind.

This was the father who had given us the living of quiet lives in familial fondness, in homes I so loved living; to plant crops in the raised beds we all had built together, and to watch the seasons come and go.

Poppa liked to tease people when they'd ask him how he was doing: "Well, both feet hit the floor at about the same time, so I must be doing just fine!" Now, those trusty old feet were no longer hitting the floor, not at the same time, nor of their own volition. Since coming home, Poppa had not gotten up or walked without our help. He could no longer put on his socks, nor close his shoes, even though we'd all been in Velcro-closing shoes for years.

Poppa has taught me much about where a woman's place was in his world. Biology notwithstanding, he taught me about how awed men are by women's constant busy-ness.

Sometimes my housekeeping would stir a memory of his life with Eva. Once upon a time, Eva had taken up sewing frocks for the women of their congregation, and Poppa had helped her sew them together, he'd enjoyed that. He would remember a cheating, slovenly cleaning girl that he and Eva had had to tolerate before firing. Sometimes, as I was about my spiderweb hunt or my dust patrol, Poppa would watch me and comment on how good I was at my work. Sometimes, when I was in a grump, I'd resent his uttering that old saw that: "A woman's work is never done." I'd mutter under my breath: *"Yes, well, if you'd try your hand at it, it might be!" Petty, petty!*

* * * * *

As he got into his car, the nurse handed us our copy of the Certificate of Impending Death.

In a gesture of fun, before we moved into our newly built home, I had framed a copy of our marriage certificate, and hung it up on the wall over our wood box. We were now in the business of practicing our marriage.

Now, I held the copy of Poppa's Impending Death Certificate, and wondered where I could put it up. Did I find one of Poppa's many old picture frames and put it in there? Where, in this tiny cabin whose walls consist of shelves and windows, could I place such a certificate? Did I take down the one we made on our first computers for Poppa's 85th birthday, or the other one we made for Father's Day this year? Did I remove the photograph of the last reunion of all ten of his brothers and sisters before they started to die off? The certificate ended up taped to the inside of the front door.

* * * * *

Today, the portable loaner hospital bed was delivered by Jim's Pharmacy. In a svelte box, no less! David and I wrestled the old poltergeist monster out of Poppa's cabin, pushing and pulling it across the gravel to its final resting place beside the garden hydrant, where it would become my work table. The hospice hadn't wanted it back.

The delivery man, with almost a magician's flourish, opened his box, and assembled the lightweight contraption in a trice. It came complete with a mini-motor and a button pad. *Ta-da!* Poppa sat the whole time fascinated, first to see us huffing and puffing with expletives galore, and then to watch the new gent perform his magic and *voilà*, a brand-spanking-new bed!

* * * * *

Later, as I drove into town to do the laundry, all I could think about was the Postmistress' hug. When I had stopped at the Post Office on Monday, to thank them for allowing a neighbor to pick up our mail, when David and Poppa had been in Seattle, Mrs. Dillard (she calls me Mrs. Brown, great affection and respect both ways) came out from behind her counter, took me in her arms and hugged me close. It was so good to lay my head on a woman's shoulder who was bigger than me, like being in the arms of the Great Goddess.

So today I was aching for that hug again, and she did. This time not letting me go, murmuring and stroking as I cried. The other workers brought me a cup of mineral water, and listened to my ramblings.

At the library, Adele, Cheryl and Dottie all took time to talk with me, comedy and sorrow. It felt again so good to be in the company of women at this time.

E-mails of the day

> *Dear Beloved Friends,*
> *Our prayers are with you through this transition.*
> *My feelings are that Lincoln could live a few days or a few years. Life and death is not up to us. What can we aspire to on this planet, a long, healthy life and a good death! Death, the ultimate lesson in letting go. It is too bad that we don't live our lives like we are going to die. Even after having lost Thomas at such a young age, I too forget that one day we are here, next day we're gone. Or worse, one day a loved-one is here, next day they are not.*
> *Death so reminded me of birth. You narrow down to what's important and real, while a transformation takes over your lives. All of birth was not especially joyful and all of death is not painful. My parents are still in their 60s, but I just visited my 88 year old grandmother this last August. It was so good to spend time with her—though I am not sure I could take care of her on the basis that you are taking care of Poppa. Even those few days of worry, med schedules, and forays in the nights, were very stressful and took a while to get over.*
> *Be kind to yourselves—you can only do the best you can, be who you are and that is enough. Lincoln is thanking his lucky stars that he has a son who is willing to take care of him and let him die a good*

natural death in the country. And thankful that he has a strong woman who loves his son, and is there for him. And as things get more real, I bet he is thankful for her direct and forthright nature.

I love you Rebecca and look forward to hearing from you soon. This is why I so love e-mail, we can stay close!

Our love and kisses, Deborah and William.

*   *   *   *   *

Dear David and Rebecca,
Make a wish before you read this poem.
Did you make a wish?
May today there be peace within.
May you trust your highest power that you are exactly where you are meant to be.
May you not forget the infinite possibilities that are born of faith.
May you use those gifts that you have received, and pass on the love that has been given to you.
May you be content knowing you are a child of God/The Creator.
Let this presence settle into your bones, and allow your soul the freedom to sing, dance and to bask in the sun.
It is there for each and every one of you.
Work like you don't need the money,
Dance like nobody's watching and
Love like you've never been hurt.
I don't know who wrote this, Artie.

*   *   *   *   *

Dear Rebecca,

I am always surprised how few people realize the sacredness of death, what an honor it is to be present. I was moved by your sharing of Poppa with me. Poppa's family has lost out on a great opportunity.

By attending to death with the same seriousness as birth, we learn how to die. We gather around to welcome new life, yet disappear when a loved-one signals it's time to die. This is why you must make space in your schedule for writing Standing The Watch. loving you, Carolyn.

Log excerpt for Day Nine of The Watch

Thursday, November 04. A powerless, stormy day.

07:00am A sleepy day for us all. David cleaned Poppa's nails. Output in his overnight bag was 400cc orange & smelly. No BMs now. Ruth says it's the morphine.

08:00 Wanted only a small bowl of cereal, *that was it, all day!* Stayed sleepy & in bed. Kept a low fire burning in his stove. we dozed & read a little, one of us over at Poppa's all day.

Poppa was pain free all day, *now that's a miracle*. Without power the oxygen machine doesn't work, soft candle light & battery lamps

Such a quietness in our lives, when the power is out.

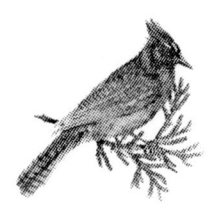

Day 9

A closer walk with Poppa

Today, we had no power as a huge Pacific Ocean storm roared over us. Dark almost all day, while we snuggled into our quiet cabins. Luckily the new loaner bed could be raised manually.

When we moved here and the huge spring storms rolled over us, tossing trees onto power lines and saturating cliff sides so that they slithered over the road, we decided to cook and heat our water with propane.

One of our first steps, after roofing and flooring Poppa's cabin, had been to wrestle the fiberglass shower stall off the back of Old Blue, and maneuver it through the gap that would be the front door. We set up the plumbing before flooring the bathroom, and then turned our attention to putting up the walls.

We lost our modesty early on as we all took spitbaths in the shower, carrying into the bathroom kettles of water heated on our wood stoves, and ladling it out for each other as we washed and rinsed. One of Poppa's jokes, which David had told me he remembered his father saying during their years in the Alaskan bush, was to remind us to spit above his head so he could run underneath it.

Later that summer, as we were building our own cabin, we also set about installing a pump beside the creek, and laying the pipes across the land to our two cabins.

We started out with a composting toilet in Poppa's bathroom. The huge contraption required electricity to run its fans, which made it quite aromatic when the power went out. Each month we paid homage to that marvel of modern engineering, by groveling in its bottom drawer where the composted wastes resided, pulling out the tray and taking it to a hole we'd dug. Three years later we graduated to a flush toilet. *Were we ever getting uptown!*

During the frequent winter power outages, we drew our washing water from a barrel under the eaves, hooked up lamps to car batteries, and quietly went on with our lives with no phone, TV, radio, pump, oxygen condenser, or the wall heater in Poppa's cabin. We would open the freezer as infrequently as possible, and it was usually chilly enough outside that our larder worked just fine. *Funny how our electricity bills never reflect these powerless days.*

* * * * *

As I was dozing today, the memory of a halcyon October day with Poppa came to mind. For weeks that summer, the weather had been warm, dry and sunny. Everyday Poppa and I had walked to the bridge where we would sit upon its retaining wall to look at the valley before us with its undulating meadows covered with brown cows and calves munching their way across the edible landscape.

That day, up near the forest edge, three mama deers and their fawns were browsing, already wearing their faded earthen color, prepared for the greenless forest underbrush of winter. Alder trees, the color of lace dipped in tea, fringed the conical conifer hillsides, their hunter green velvet pile upon the hips of the Earth. Beyond glowed the great westering sun, casting ripe autumnal hues.

Poppa and I had sat there awhile with Buddy-dog beside us, bored until he curled up behind Poppa's legs for a nap. We had relaxed in the fresh fall air and stared at the dying-away of so many brilliant summer days. Days tending a picture-book garden with sturdy raised beds crowned with a glory of tomatoes, the result of Poppa's labors. He would spend ages each day, leaning on his cane with one hand while, with the other he meticulously pollinated each and every flower. He had made a brush from a feather a bird had given him, and whittled a cedar stick from our kindling boxes. In another bed was a swatch of healthy bright leaves of the Swiss Chard, which we loved steamed. Another bed was filled with four kinds of lettuce, eager with their tasty offerings. Poppa and I would peer over it as he selected the leaves for our salads, and I picked and placed them into the wicker basket.

On this particular day, as we headed home with the sun warming our backs, masses of orange and black caterpillars had been crawling hither and yon across the road. We counted until we lost count. I commented on the imagery of us being like caterpillars, and passing through the Veil of Death to become butterflies in heaven.

"Can't...they don't have souls." Poppa had murmured breathlessly.

"Who don't?" I queried confused.

"Them."

"The caterpillars?"

"Yes."

"How do you know? What a strange thing to think," quoth I, both curious and amused. Long silence as we plodded on, our shadows before us and autumn light glowing on trees, road, leaves and the last apples in an orchard. Then Poppa spoke of the Vision he'd had just after he was Saved, and was bothered about his mother's relationship to the Lord.

As we walked in the warmth, the scents of fall filling the air and no traffic on the road, this old stumbling man, who believed caterpillars had no souls, told me of seeing his mother in one of her print dresses, she favored print dresses, coming down a hill, hip high in grasses, smiling and waving to him. He guessed she was all right with the Lord.

We had walked on a few more paces when I commented: "What a lovely, lovely vision, Poppa."

"Yes, it is."

"Very healing."

"I found it so."

"Warms the heart."

"That it does."

And on we had stumbled to our home, where David had dinner waiting for us.

Log excerpt for Day Ten of The Watch

Friday, November 05
07:00am Awake, no "Good morning, Sweetheart!" today. Wanted to go to his recliner, only cornflakes & milk.
09:00 Hungry again. Wanted a soft-boiled egg, a taste of ham & half a slice of toast. Didn't eat much of it though.
09:20 Took some pain medications. Threw up. Changed patch. Drank a little water. *I can't stand this!* He's been vomiting consistently since the change in pain meds.
Noon Tried Rx drink. Threw up. Didn't want water. He looks so sad & wan. Sat with him quietly, holding his hand. Doesn't want the TV on. Loves having the picnic table outside his window so he can watch the chipmunks & blue jays.
01:15 Tried a little milk. Threw up, curdled. *I want to howl!*
02:00 Moved back to bed. Threw up. Poor feller looks so miserable. I bet his esophagus is sore. Lying down is the only comfortable place.
02:15 Chest pain. 1 nitro tab. *Here we go!*
03:00 More pain. 2 drops of morphine Rx as per doc.
04:00 More pain in back of neck. Changed position.
04:45 Chest pain. 1 more nitro tab.
04:50 Still 50% pain. 3rd nitro tab. Fell asleep. The cannula for the oxygen irritates him, he keeps rubbing his nose, pushing the tubes around. That throbbing machine gives me a headache.
05:30 Time to change the catheter. Urine: 350cc & cloudy, almost opaque. David quietly performed the rit-

ual & I cleaned the bag & hung it to dry. Cleaned up the bathroom. *What a smell of vomit*!

09:00 Poppa asleep. I collapse in bed. David reads in his chair.

Today was a very bad day. I hated almost every minute of it!

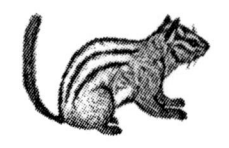

Day 10

Uphill and into the wind

"One thing that comes out in myths...is that at the bottom of the abyss comes the voice of salvation. The black moment is...when the real message of transformation...comes [to] light."
Joseph Campbell, *The Power of Myth*

This dying isn't all adventure. It's the worst kind of waiting. I get flushes of embarrassment when I hear that little voice in my head saying: *"Piss or get off the pot!"* I remember one weekend when my father was dying. We were not allowed to watch TV during the day unless it was a national emergency; nor listen to the radio; ditto my record player. I'd read about all I could and my mother had told me to stop typing as the noise might bother Father. In frustration I had prostrated myself on my bed, crying and heard that little voice in my head hiss: *"Die or get up and live!"* I was racked with remorse that such a thought could find life in my mind.

*　　*　　*　　*　　*

As an adopted child coming up behind three brothers, two of whom were our parents' offspring, observing and watching the genetic, kinetic heritage between family members, has been a motif in my life.

I never had relatives to match myself up to so, until I had my own children, I felt unattached to anyone, a mirror without reflection. I have always secretly stared at families to see how the children looked like their parents, their siblings and their cousins. When I looked at our history books, I'd see the inherited features of the monarchs down the centuries. I'd notice the similarities of sisters at my schools and then, on Parents Day, I'd glimpse their mothers, their mothers' sisters and, if I was lucky, their grandmothers.

So, as is my wont, when I came face-to-face with David's father, I noticed the breadth of chest, set of shoulders, eyebrows and hands. Poppa's were huge, gnarled, heavily veined, with liver spots, and an index finger with a bent top joint, yet both father and son's hands were distinctly similar.

While Poppa had a full head of hair, Eva's father had had male pattern baldness, which David inherited. When I met Poppa, his hair was thick, cut severely short and white-walled around his ears. He was also clean shaven. Early in our homesteading he had, for about two years, decided to grow a beard for the first time in his life. He also let his hair grow long until, on our way home from Port Angeles one afternoon, as we were passing a log cabin that sported a barber's pole, he suddenly asked us to stop there. When he came back out and settled into his seat, Buddy-dog was all of a-tremble with confusion. Sniffing and licking Poppa, grunting in his particular way of questioning. Poppa got quite a kick out of that!

Whereas my beloved, who is going bald, has sported a fine moustache and a resplendent beard most of his life.

Poppa had a stooped back, which I hadn't noticed that first time I saw him sitting in the booth at breakfast. It was only when he walked off to his pick up truck across the parking lot, that I saw it. David told me his dad's back had always been bent, the result of holding the reins of the plow since he was five years old. I was astonished that I had just met someone who had actually worked a horse-drawn plow. A chiropractor we all frequented, knew well enough to leave alone that question mark in his spine. I'm sure that posture had a lot to do with Poppa's acid reflux problems, as his stomach was permanently squashed.

I was fascinated to see how an adult son and father interacted. Sometimes they actually held conversations. When they were working together in their refinishing shop, they talked about instructions, and how things came apart and went back together. Sometimes the son chided the father for a faulty memory. Sometimes the father remembered something his son had not known.

I noticed that Poppa never talked about his missionary years. *Not that I wanted to hear any preaching!* I was simply curious about such an absence in Poppa's stories. When I asked David about it, he told me that when his father had come to live with him, he had laid down the law about his father eternally bending his ear about religion.

David's parents had groomed him to be a preacher, and their son had excelled. As David grew to manhood in the Reservations of the South West, this son of two preachers had also been a student of a Harvard-educated Blessing

Way Singer of the Dine' (Navajo) People. At the same time in his life, David had gone on his Vision Quest and been ordained as a Christian minister. It was the military that rescued him from this double life, sending him, as a military analyst, all over the world and eventually to Viet Nam. *Out of the frying pan, into the fire!*

Sometimes Poppa got hold of a story, and there we were until it ended. A gem of a memory, told in his gravelly drawl. This old feller knew well how to tell a story. He should have had umpteen grandchildren at his knees! In the beginning I would listen, fascinated. David had heard them all, many, many times.

Each year at the end of winter, when we'd drive by a certain bog along the road where the yellow hoods of the Skunk Cabbages were visible, out would come Poppa's story of how his city bride had urged him to pick a bouquet of those colorful, wild plants.

"You don't want me to do that!" Poppa would recount with a chuckle.

"Yes, yes I do!" His new bride had retorted, and so he had trod through the swamp and picked her a bouquet. When he proffered it to her, she had grabbed it with glee and buried her unsuspecting nose into the bright blossoms.

At this point in the story, Poppa's voice would be throbbing with laughter. "Dang it, if she didn't shriek like a chicken chased by a fox!" In an instant she had thrown the bouquet out the window of their pickup, weeping at the stench which she could not scour off her hands.

As Poppa began to rapidly ripen, his memories slithered one into the other and he'd ramble on for ages, segueing from story to story as something would jog a memory. Sometimes the two-hour drive to Port Angeles would be a marathon of murmurings, recounted to Buddy-dog as he laid his head on his master's lap, with soulful eyes upraised, drinking it all in.

One of the things the harried nurses in the hospitals always commented on, was Poppa's storytelling, and the images he evoked of another time and place. Women are innately polite, we wait until a person stops talking, before we say or do something. Like the nurses, I too had to learn to become impolite, and interrupt Poppa's stories so I could do my duty.

He should have had a lodge of brothers with whom he could exchange stories. When our neighbor men would come out of the woods to feast with us at Thanksgiving, he would remain silent for ages and then, finding a moment, he'd dive in. That was when everyone sat back in their chairs, lit up their smokes, put wood in the stove, and let him take us away. He should have had a tribe of great-grandsons at his knees!

* * * * *

We'd been weepy and weary today. I had just unpacked the laundry when Poppa threw up again. His urine was cloudy when I emptied the bag. We had managed to get him back to bed, he does so love sitting in his recliner, watching the forest and the weather. He can't make his legs move much, the connections seemed to be going. He had refused most food and drink and, of course, all his medications, except those for the pain when it comes.

The home health nurses reminded us they were on call, day and night, for us when we were worried. It was his throwing up after a couple of sips of water. There was nothing for him to vomit, a sip of milk and up it came!

He'd been resting comfortably and for the first time we had to use the morphine for the pain. The nurses calmly explained about the systems beginning to shut down, and for us to expect the end soon. *Whatever soon means!*

David recalled Poppa saying he'd been born in a thunder and lightening storm in Kansas, and now it was gently raining, setting the night a-glistening. Poppa's cabin was snug and warm, with the string of Christmas lights he so loved, glowing around his bathroom door, and his beloved Buddy-dog asleep under the bed.

Last night Poppadum had the first totally pain-free night in two months, amazing! All three of us got six solid hours of sleep. I surfaced now and again, expecting to hear the alarm chimes ringing. Was rather expecting to greet a cadaver when I walked in this morning. Instead I met a bright eyed, chipper, joking, hungry old feller!

"Good morning, Sweetheart!"

"Good morning, Poppa!"

We go in bouts of gallows humor, snuffling fear, sadness and just plain "let's get the job done!" In discussing these sorts of things, Poppa's epitaph was going to be: Here Lies A Good Man. I thought it perfect.

Buddy-dog began having seizures the day after Poppa got home. He has been miserable, torn between hiding out under Poppa's bed and dashing out for a sniff of fresh air. Every other day, as one of us tended to Poppa, the other cared for Buddy-dog, murmuring to him as he convulsed, his eyes glazed, his breathing shallow, his body trembling. We found that hard rubbing on his chest really helped, as well as simply getting down on the floor and being right there in his face, touching him, talking to him. Those seizures last only a few minutes, after which he's thirsty and shaky and clingy. Then he just has to go outside. Right now? "Woof! woof!"

We're so tired. Poppa's sleeping at last and so shall I. David's dozing in his chair. Midnight and all is well, sort of, maybe. How long, Mother Spider, how long? Not that I want Poppa to leave, mind you! How fast we insist life be lived.

E-mails of the day

> Rebecca,
> Don't worry, there's plenty of time for phone calls.
> I like the epitaph. Nice and simple and to the point, saying it all. Bean counters must be a term you brought over the waters with you. You are so poetic in your articulation. Hope you're getting another night's worth of good sleep while I write this and wonder why I myself am not snuggling under covers.
> Good night and lots of love, Faina

*   *   *   *   *

> Rebecca, I've been wondering how Poppa was doing. Thanks for letting me know. I know this is an exhausting time for all of you and, as you said, a time to reflect on our own mortality. We have had several deaths recently of two favorite uncles...both very sudden. We have had many of the same discussions that I believe you and David are having now.
> I really chuckled over your hospital bed story. Pretty eerie!!

I trust that Poppa will be comfortable during his last days. I know you and David will do everything possible to make this possible.
Thinking of you, Love, Jane and Keith.

   * * * * *

Thanks Rebecca, great bed story, just what we needed, some good chuckles.
Saying prayers for y'all. Artie.

Log excerpt for Day Eleven of The Watch

Saturday, November 06.
04:10am Groggy with sleep, Poppa said: "...take this thing out of my nose." We detached the cannula. Then "...can't sleep with all that racket." Turned off the condenser.
07:00 Chest pains again. 2 drops morphine.
07:15 Took the patch off as we wiped him down with alcohol. Heels are red as too his shoulder blades & hump. Urine out: 600cc cloudy. What a kerfuffle over the sterile water! The pharmacist says it's used in making illegal drugs, that's why you have to have an Rx for it. My, are we out of the loop!
08:00 Pain. 2 drops morphine. *What prayers are there for this pain?*
08:20 Pain. 1 drop.
08:40 Still bad pain. 2 more drops. New nitro patch.
09:10 Called HH nurse: none of the above is relieving the pain.
09:20 In half tsp water, dissolve 1 anxiety pill w/2 drops morphine. *Another little lesson in chemistry*.
09:25 50% pain gone. *Ah, the grimace is leaving!*
09:32 Still 25% of pain. That crease of pain on his brow is still there.
09:38 Still 25% of pain. 2 more drops. Lips & tongue exploring.
10:45 "...when are we going to eat?" Dry mouth. Sipped 75cc of water. Eyes open, vague & bright. Wanted Rx drink, sipped 50cc. Slept.
02:00pm Awoke. Wanted a bed bath. Some pain. Repeated dosage.

06:00 Chest pain & lower throat now. Repeated dosage. New patch.

08:45 1 more drop. No water.

09:20 Sweaty & miserable, jerking & muttering.

10:20 SEVERE PAIN! Given 4 drops. Sweating & groaning.

10:25 NO RELIEF! 4 more drops. NO RELIEF AT ALL!

10:39 Pain increased. David finally read the package insert. It says to give more than what the doctor ordered & more often.

10:40 Called home health nurse. Give 2 mashed-up anxiety pills. 2nd call to discuss meds & relieve our anxiety. Still groaning & grimacing.

10:55 Still severe pain. More morphine drops.

11:08 Pain down 55%. Home health nurse called us back. "You're doing just fine, go with the flow. The pain relief will come."

11:25 Home health nurse called to check on progress. Suggested he get back on oxygen & to give him nitro tabs in the next bout. *There's going to be more?*

11:30 1 nitro. He agreed to be connected back up to oxygen. On comes that hissing, roaring motor & the whole cabin throbs. Hollow floors! Sounds like a song title.

11:35 1 more nitro. Slowly, slowly the grimacing evaporates.

Hurry up! Hurry up with everything. Here we are, in slow motion; one breath at a time.

Breathe in, breathe out.

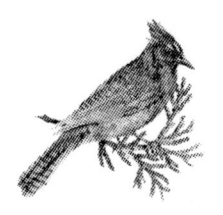

Day 11

A nickel's worth of five dollar bills

David was the only child of Lincoln and Eva's marriage, and in my family, I was the youngest and only daughter. Together in this home death, we walk side-by-side in step, like horses in harness pulling Poppa's wagon. There is no time for socialization, and we don't have anything anyone wants to hear. Home deathing can be a conversation stopper. We have resisted going to town as neither of us wants to leave, just in case.

No one calls, no one drops by. Where are the women with the vittles and the men with the prayers? Is that what society has lost? Had we joined Poppa's church with him, would we now be surrounded by fellow congregants? Were we to live closer to town, would we be visited more often? *Would we want it?*

Or is Standing The Watch of death something to be shunned? A time to be absent? Who has the time to waste, nowadays, in waiting for someone to die? We put our animals down in the blink of an eye, why not ourselves? We put our criminals to death with strange ceremonies while a host of people watch. *What's wrong with dying at home?*

Or is it that we've decided dying is a failure? The impression I got from my mother's behavior, after my father's death, was how dared he go die on her? How dared he make her a widow? Her not talking about him or his dying before, during or after, perplexed me. It was that silence that scared me. Being separated from the event, relegated to a problem that had to be sent away while the serious ceremony was happening, made dying, for me, a frightening mystery. Did my mother sit by her husband's side as the sands of his life trickled through his hourglass? Did she stand beside him as he drew his last breath and exhaled out of this world?

We have been pulling in the traces of our marriage, a husband and wife tending to the dying of the Elder in our clan. Watching and waiting. Murmuring and hugging. Who remembers to eat? Who remembers our own body functions? Legs and backs ache. We dare not take our own pain pills for fear of falling into a deep sleep when we're most needed.

What a feeling of abandonment. Only my e-mail friends are there. People gush about coming out to help us and do not arrive. People ask if there's anything they can do and a slew of answers slither through my brain, by-passing my tongue. Bring us food? Spell us while we catch some shut-eye? Relieve us for a day—to do what? It all seems too petty.

Brother Death has come for a visit. Where once we thought we had months, now we have only days, maybe hours. It behooves us to stay on The Watch, in service, taking care of the business at hand; completing each bout of pain, with as much calm as we can. Heck, we're so tired, neither of us could get frantic even if we wanted to!

I often wondered at David's feelings about watching his father die. The memories of his boyhood, to this man's fatherhood. A child conceived after the Second World War to a man born before the First. What worlds apart! Poppa is not the first man my husband has seen die. As a Viet Nam Veteran in the field, he has seen his share of dying. As an Alaskan Big Game Guide, he has made his share of death. We talk and talk—when we're not napping or tending Poppa.

And me, what do I see as I watch this Old Soul readying to return from whence it came? I watch the once lively body, moving reflexively rather than intentionally. Meeting Poppa only a few years ago, I did not know him when he was hale and hearty. I keep seeing the raising of a baby, as if played backwards.

Is it scary? Not really. The fear is more that I shall do something wrong. That I will cause him more pain and discomfort. That someone will call me on the carpet for making a mistake. That's an old, old knee-jerk reaction. Perhaps it's a woman's thing, living in a man's world where they have laid out all the rules and rituals to life.

Now, as we are about the purpose of Standing The Watch as our elder prepares to leave us, I see images of thousands of years-old flowers scattered in a grave in a cave. How far away from that kind of dying have we moved! Would I, for a moment, wish Poppa in the care of strangers in a strange place? No! This is what Spirit has given us to do, at this time, in this place. What else would we be doing?

Just as in birth, death offers us a time to stop our world and watch and listen, to be in the moment, to live in the very pulse of life.

One moment we breathe, and the next we are gone. Just like that!

*   *   *   *   *

And so we stood The Watch together, my husband and I. And in that aloneness, our marriage was more alive and kicking than had we been traipsing off to a distant place to be relegated to spectators. Perhaps that, of all our rejections of public facilities for birthing and dying, was what we objected to the most—being cast as an audience, rather than in supporting roles.

Death comes to us all. No one gets out of Life alive and I think about my own dying, about the dying of my husband, my children, my father so long ago and the mother of my childhood so far away, and I wonder about what being alive means.

E-mails of the day

> Reb and David...you were so in my thoughts today, I glanced thru your e-Mail this morning on my way out the door.
>
> What a grand service you are doing for Papa, and for yourselves too, for midwifing this transition can be as grand as any birthing.
>
> I was glad to hear they have a pain cocktail for Papa, and he's able to take it still. If it gets to the point where he can't swallow, they do have patches that can be put on and absorbed thru the skin.

One thing I want to mention is that oftentimes the patient may be semi-comatose and it looks like things are coming to an end when they will suddenly rally for a short lucid time. It's almost as if they have finished their business between the worlds and decided to come back for a final goodbye. It can be a real precious bit of time.
love to you all....RR

*   *   *   *   *

Dearest friend,
I could feel the heaviness of your environment and ish I had more support to offer. I'm not sure if I could take care of another person again. Think I've had my fill of care taking. Time to be taken care of. It's been my experience for years that the ones with the least amount seem to give the most.

Ok, my dear, keep on keeping on and right here, always on the other side of cyberspace, being there for you in whatever limited way I can, is me, Faina.

Log excerpt for Day Twelve of The Watch

Sunday, November 07

01:00pm Returned from laundry, kissed Poppa hello & put away the linens. Suddenly, Poppa's hand is flailing at the alarm button: "...a little pain." Changed nitro patch.

02:45 "...a little pain" again. I nitro tab + ice chips. Deep sleep.

03:50 Woke grimacing, restless. Anxiety pills crushed in water.

06:38 Alarm chimes. Pain. Can't describe it. Morphine+1 nitro.

06:45 Still pain. Called HH nurses. Give more morphine.

07:00 Any pain? Handshake. Changed pj top & pad. Dry heaves.

09:30 Alarm chimes. Pain. 1 nitro. Sweating again. 250cc out.

09:35 50% pain reduced. He doesn't respond. Can't get another tab under his tongue.

09:37 2 calmers+morphine as per nurse. *I could do with a couple of calmers!*

10:00pm Sleeping.

Breathe in, breathe out.

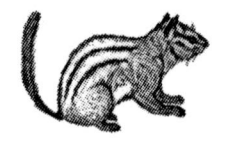

Day 12

Famous last words

What an up and down day. Glad to get away and glad to come home. Haven't watched TV in days, just quiet music playing. Reading seems the only way David and I can relax.

I drove into town today to do the laundry. Old habits die hard. For the past six years that is what I've done on Sundays. My cleanliness next to godliness routine. Dropping Poppa off at his church, and then driving down that swooping long hill to the bay and the little village we call town, to meander through its back street to the laundromat in the trailer park.

Today, as I swept past the church, its parking lot chock-a-block with congregants' cars, I imagined entering their chapel and giving them what-for as they all sit in their weekly worship while their oldest congregant lies dying. Their mind set seems so alien. I think back on the Catholic priests and Jewish rabbis I have known, and how they'd wrap themselves up into the intimate details of dying. I know I'll not be able to look that pastor in the face again.

When I first took Poppa to that church at his request, they tried to seduce me in. Oh, everso welcoming, everso charming. The women and men in their Sunday Best, all trolling, eager to retrieve a lost soul. No one bothered to ask me if I felt lost. Even Poppa, for a couple of years as he got out of our minivan heading for the chapel, would wistfully invite me to postpone my washing and partake of their spiritual feast.

I did not get their religious point of view, especially about birthdays and Christmas, which they ignored. What a slap in the face of motherhood, and the celebration of childhood and this grand adventure we call Life! For too many years, I have been made to feel like a second-class human by the religions of men. Out of our wombs they come, and then spend the rest of their lives hacking women to pieces.

I was in such a rage today at the laundry, it was just as well no one was there. Each load of Poppa's vomitous towels and jammies was a prayer, an exhortation and yes, a bit of a curse. I imagined dunking the pastor and his sweet-smiling wife into the washing machine and scouring away their platitudes. I imagined tossing the congregants into the dryers and willing their sorry little souls into fluffed-up, absorbent Cosmic compassion.

While I waited for the cycles to complete, I stared up at the forested hills in the misty, pouring rain and thought about dying; about exiting this life; about leaving it all behind and heading off into places unknown. They talk about an after life as if it is a carrot held before us to urge us on through some miserable chore. They talk about their relationship with their Lord. *What gives with that in a democracy?* I, who have lived in a society where lords abound, know from aristocracy and servanthood; know these sorry little souls will have quite a jolt when they come into the presence of their expectations!

Or are heaven and hell, gods and prophets merely figments of our imaginations? Wet dreams of our souls yearning for comfort? Is their version of spiritual reality any better, any more valid than mine? Who's to say Mother Spider isn't at The Center? Who's ever come back and told us what's ahead? Who's got the monopoly on spiritual rightness?

With each item I pulled from the dryers and tossed upon the folding table, I thought about a person's life. How we remember them. How we're exhorted to speak no ill of the dead, only to remember the good. Poppa lived by a slew of taboos. Asking him a direct question often deteriorated into an eternally looping contest, humor notwithstanding! It was a struggle to get him to say yes or no, with respect to his wants and needs. For two summers he had eaten steamed Brussels sprouts (which I relish!), before finally murmuring that he didn't care for them. The only way he knew how to get his way, was to passively wait you out, sitting like a bump on a log, until you gave up. When he aired his opinion about something social, it was often archaic racism, or ignorance. So Poppa could be a crabby old man, so what? He knew what he knew, and he walked his walk. He stayed in the traces long after most folks had kicked over them and headed for the happy playgrounds of retirement.

I was angry as I folded umpteen towels and sheets. And I was frightened about life after Poppa's death. What would we do? How would we earn our keep? I thought of my mother, and the months after her husband's death, and realized what I had not before understood. My mother had been frightened. After thirty years of marriage, suddenly she had to fend for herself. She had masked that fear with fury, much of which splattered over me as the last of the children still at home.

Laundry done and loaded, I drove in a hurry to the county park to pee. Rebelling against dashing home to relieve my husband, and postponing the moment when I must drive past that damn church again, I leashed Buddy-dog for a hard, fast walk along the beach.

There, Sister Sea sang to me; soothing me with her susurrant songs, rinsing away my rage. Tears poured for an old man who had devoted half his 89 years to bringing the word of his salvation to the heathens, and when it comes time for him to die, not one of his fellow spiritual brothers and sisters will come near him!

Sister Sea sang to me her songs of reconciliation, of grief and fear. I bent for a scoop of her salty tears, and made the gestures of homage and recognition. Tasting her saltiness and smelling her sweet perfume. Poor Buddy-dog shivered and cowed beside me. This was not his idea of a fun run. We stumbled back across the pebbles, slipping and sliding until we stepped on solid ground and faced the graceful arching bridge that spanned the outlet of the Clallam River. Crossing the Rubicon. Even this we have changed in our arrogance. 'Sklallam was what the First People called this area; much too complicated for our Western tongues! I was furious with everyone as I stomped through the naked alder grove, back to the warmth of my beloved minivan, and turned her around to head for home.

Wait, I had to do some shopping! With my basket of necessaries, I approached the checkout stand and there, Cosmically, was Karen. When she saw me weepy and angry, she came around and even though I was wet and cold, she enfolded me in a long hug. Murmuring and stroking me as if I were a lost child. I bawled.

That done, we grinned and she checked me out and loaded up my groceries. I gave Buddy-dog his much-earned stick of jerky, and headed home. So relieved was I that it wasn't until I slowed down for the dead man's curves, that I realized I'd passed the church without noticing. In a lighter mood, I turned onto our road for the twelve-mile run through valleys and hills, driving deep into the dripping rainforest.

At home again, in the warmth of our cabins with their bright lights, I toweled Buddy-dog dry and gave my welcoming husband a long wet hug. Together we put away the freshly laundered linens. We were family once again, for as long as it was to be.

As David was helping Poppa settle for the evening, Poppa spoke:

"Son, I feel like I'm going downhill fast!" His son had replied, as he stroked his father's hand.

"Maybe, Poppa, you're really going up hill!" And with that Poppa laid back and sighed.

*   *   *   *   *

Dear All,

Poppa seems to be resting comfortably. No food or drink for 2 days and slips in and out of deep sleep. Had to use the morphine full strength last night for first time.

He asks me all kinds of questions out of the blue. I'm just giving the best answers I can at the moment and holding his hand w/a few ice chips to moisten his mouth, won't take water.

Rebecca and I are holding up fairly well. Short naps and we spell each other. Things are getting quieter and we find that hugs are spontaneous things that happen as we pass. Thoughts are often rambling scrambles after some long lost moment.

Time marches on as we shades stand on the curb and watch the procession go by. Reality becomes distant and values shift with each passing minute.

Three days ago is so far in the past and my childhood only yesterday. Each gentle return squeeze of his hand evokes powerful mental flashes of forgotten landscapes. Frozen film that is so vivid, so rich and deep that I wonder how I ever forgot that particular moment.

Later, Love, David

Log excerpt for the Last Day of The Watch

Monday, November 08
12:05am Sleeping? Any pain? "No." Learning the language of the physical. We speak & Poppa gestures with his whole body.
01:20 Pain. 1 nitro pill which he swallowed instead of letting dissolve under his tongue. *How could he do anything else?*
01:24 2nd nitro. No relief. Just the grimace & gripping hands.
01:29: Rx drops, dripped into Poppa's mouth over his dry lips.
01:37 Relief. No response from him now.
02:05 Sleeping. & so do we in garden chairs beside his bed.
04:30am Now Poppa has a frown. Dripped ice chips on his lips. He actually cleared his throat. Gave a faint nod to our question about pain. David mixed another cocktail.
06:30 Sleeping & so were we
08:00 Took a drop of water. Soothed his feet w/alcohol swab.
11:00 The HH nurse arrives. She strokes our shoulders & tells us we're doing well & that it will be soon. Watches David change the nitro patch.
11:28 Still in pain; she suggests more Rx drops. Sleeping.
Noon HH nurse leaves, reminds us to call when things change.
12:45 More pain. More drops.

01:43 Suddenly his hand rises up & pulls the oxygen cannula out. Breathing becomes varied. I turn off the oxygen condenser.

01:55 Deeply non-responsive. Long exhalations.

02:08 Deep frown. Facial grimaces. Extremities jerking. Read Psalms from his Bible. Seemed to relax him.

02:15 Frown gone. Legs spasm less. Breathing more even.

03:26pm Took a deep breath, exhaled & did not breathe again.

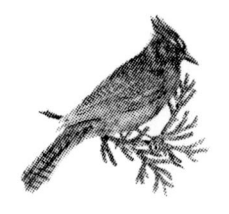

Day 13

He restoreth my soul

Psalm 23

These last days and nights have been marked only by light and dark, rain or sun, whether the stoves needed wood, whether we were awake or asleep. Every other day a home health nurse arrived to monitor our efforts, to give us information, and to chart Poppa's progress toward his inevitable transformation.

Sometimes we thought about food, although neither of us was hungry. Poppa was no longer consuming anything other than occasional ice chips melted on his lips.

Even though it was a winter day, Poppa's cabin glowed. There was a peace and a quietness as we waited, on each side of Poppa's bed, listening to this old feller breathing, watching him, stroking and murmuring now and again of our love, our gratitude and how his job here on earth was done.

There was no rigid grimace on his beloved face, for he no longer felt any pain. Poppa was going quietly and without hindrance, toward his departure. One time his hand rose up and pulled the cannula out, his breathing became varied. I turned off the noisy machine. Poppa became deeply non-responsive.

Breathe in, breathe out.

We stood beside our Poppa, stroking his gnarled hands, smoothing his brow and short grey hair. We kissed his cheeks on which only a fuzz had grown in the past week, murmured our love and thanks, and waited.

Breathe in. Breathe out.

There was nowhere more important to be, nothing more important to do. Light glowed, he glowed. Sounds from outside dissolved with the crackle of the wood stove, with Buddy-dog chasing something in his sleep on his blankets under the bed. My beloved husband's presence, watching over his father's dying, filled my universe.

Sometime in that waiting, I heard a call in my mind to read the Scriptures and I let go Poppa's hand, crossed the cabin to pull out his worn Bible from the bag I'd sewn so many years ago so that on Sundays, he could carry his sacred text and have his hands free for his walking sticks.

The Book fell open in my hands at the Psalms, and I simply began reading the ones to which my eyes were directed. Those well-marked, well-known poems from the ancients in that lyrical language, flowed from my tongue and my memory. When I'd come upon the fire and brimstone, retribution and sinning stuff, I'd simply skip over to the next paean of faith, joy and gratitude.

I held Poppa's hand as I read, stroking slowly with my thumb and out of the corner of my eye I could see this man's son, my helpmate and friend, holding his father's hand and listening to the sacred words, at peace with the process, entirely in the moment, resting and remembering.

Poppa's entire body seemed to sigh as he heard those familiar words, his shaking hand pulsed in mine, a pinkness suffused him, almost a smile upon his lips. On and on his valiant heart labored, and his great lungs breathed in, breathed out.

At the end of a gentle verse, I sensed it was done and closed his Bible against my chest, standing silent, in that home Poppa had helped build, where his Buddy-dog lived and the blue jays hopped over the conical roof; where the wall clock tick-tocked on and a logging truck or a plane or perhaps a storm rumbled outside. I looked out of the window above Poppa's bed and saw a fading winter day, with rain on its way; and the quietness of the moment, of the here and now was simply to be lived.

Breathe in, breathe out.

So the sound of my stomach growling seemed oddly loud, and when David's also grumbled, suddenly I knew we were hungry. I couldn't remember when we had last eaten. Time to break our fast. I kissed Poppa's hand, his cheek and brow and told him where I am going and murmured again how I have loved him. I hugged and kissed my husband and left him at his father's side.

Breathe in, breathe out.

As I returned from fixing salads, David came out of Poppa's door. We met on the porch and it was then that I noticed how dark were the circles under his eyes, how tired and yet contented was this big man of mine.

"He's gone," he murmured, "I'd just come back in from a leak and a smoke, and had just picked up his hand again, and told him I was back, when he took one deep breath and let it out, and didn't breathe again."

I stepped into my husband's waiting arms and we hugged and sighed.

It was done and Poppa had returned to his Maker. Lincoln was at last with his Lord and Savior, his innings was over, his life's course run. What stories he now takes back to the Source; what reunions are in progress!

It was done! Poppa had taken his last earthly breath and left the building.

When I entered Poppa's cabin, I could feel the change, see the glow rising up. I went to my side of his bed, took up his hand and kissed it for the last time, stroked his hair for the last time, kissed his cheek for the last time. I looked upon the face of this wise old feller, looked hard at the look of Death. How still was his bag of bones. I kept expecting that massive chest to rise again, and my lungs ached for want of his breathing.

Together we washed our father's feet, hands and face with the soft creek water. David performed his last rite of disconnecting the catheter tube and pulling off the condom. I poured the dregs of Poppa's life out into the toilet. It was only when I turned to perform my ritual of cleansing and disinfecting, readying it for its next use, that I realized I didn't need to anymore. This time the bag would be burned. Because of the morphine there had been a plug in Poppa's bowels for days, he hadn't eaten anything anyway. So this dear Old Soul taught us one more lesson about the dignity of dying and a cleanliness so close to godliness.

Back at Poppa's bed, David showed me the Ritual of Laying Out the Dead. Gently washing and dressing him in his best pjs. With ribbons I'd set aside just for this purpose, we tied closed his jaw; tied together his feet, so very like his son's. Before tying together his hands, we put the special piece of wood Poppa had whittled for slipping through Buddy-dog's leash handle so that his numbed fingers could keep a firmer grip.

We quietly spoke to Poppa's Spirit as we took care, for the final time, of his earthly remains, and I sang songs for his departure, while Buddy-dog slept beneath the bed. David had turned off the heater, opened the door for Poppa's Spirit, as his tradition required; letting in cool, clean, moist air.

By the time David called the funeral home from our cabin, it was raining in earnest and getting dark. We had been told that were we to call after 5pm, they would not be able to collect the remains until the next morning, unless we paid an overtime surcharge.

Once again this frugal father had taken care of his children. The driver said he would start out momentarily; he knew his way as he had often driven to the lake for camping and fishing with his sons. In fact, he had been there the previous week, and thought about stopping off to meet us. He said he hadn't wanted to disturb us. He advised us it would be well over two hours before he got there. We let him know we'd be standing at the end of our driveway with flashlights.

We called around to our neighbors. Some thanked us for letting them know; others asked if we needed them there; one was not yet back from work so I left a message on her machine.

It was this neighbor, Pam Carlson, who came trotting up the rain-slicked road in the dark an hour later, to give us watery hugs. Because we couldn't remain indoors, we'd been standing out in the storm at the end of our driveway. When I asked if she'd like to see Poppa, she immediately agreed. I led her into Poppa's darkened and chilly cabin, for we'd let the fire go out and had turned out all the lights, except for a votive candle I had lit when we began to lay our Poppa out.

Now, I noticed how yellow the hue of Poppa's flesh had become. Now there is no pinkish bloom. Now the stern visage seemed gaunt and empty. The glow had gone from the cabin, as if Poppa's Spirit had indeed left the building, and all that remained was the remains. So this, at last, was Death. All my wondering since I was fifteen had been addressed. I felt as if I was in a resonating place of peace. *Perhaps it was only exhaustion!*

Pam inspected Poppa's Laying in State and commended us. She spoke about how peaceful Poppa looked. Being a hospital nurse, she said, didn't often allow her to witness an easy death, an expected death, a gentle death. This was very beautiful and she thanked us for this opportunity. Naturally, we were flooded with tears of validation.

Around six o'clock, we three were again standing in our hats and ponchos, at the end of our driveway, in the dark of a now windy rainstorm. After the commute of friends honking as they drove home, we noticed a vehicle's headlights slowly coming toward us and we waved our flashlights. Pam and I sloshed back to Poppa's cabin, and turned on all the inside and outside lights, and David waved in the backing minivan.

Because of the rain and the gravel path, the Bodyman hurriedly carried in the gurney between the balustrades we had built years ago after Poppa had toppled one unsteady afternoon. With four adults, a gurney, a hospital bed, table and an oxygen condenser, that little cabin was crowded! The Bodyman was trying to be solemn and polite as we bumped into each other when suddenly a Poppa-like joke popped out of David's mouth. The Bodyman, seeing it was all right, relaxed and started talking us through the next steps.

When he had Poppa's bag of bones ready to be lifted into the body bag on the gurney, he murmured. "This is one big feller!" And yes, Poppa had been a massively made man, retaining breadth of chest and shoulder all his livelong days.

With Pam and me on one side, and David and the Bodyman on the other, we lifted the body into the bag and with a flourish, the zipper was drawn. Done! A few forms to sign and he'd be on his way. I thought to let him know, seeing as how Poppa had requested cremation, that there would be two metal knee replacements among the ashes, and he took due note of that.

Then we wrestled the gurney along the gravel path, loaded it into the van, and with a cheery farewell, the Bodyman drove off into the dark and stormy night.

All this time, Buddy-dog had not moved from under Poppa's bed. When that minivan's motor started up and it began to roll, he came skittering out, sniffing and sneezing, whining and barking. Suddenly every dog in the valley was joining in, and Poppa was escorted off with a canine chorus.

Pam hugged us and trotted home and suddenly, there at the end of the driveway, we were standing in the rain and wind, done, spent. We gathered up Buddy-dog's blankets and food bowl, turned out all the lights, and finally closed Poppa's cabin.

We made our way to our home where we stoked up the stove, talked to and caress a lost dog, and sat in our chairs. *What on earth were we supposed to do now?*

*   *   *   *   *

Dear Friends,
At 3:26pm PST Poppa took a deep breath and left for parts unknown.

I'm in the process of taking care of the garment left behind.

Rebecca and I are OK. Now life goes on in this plane for us, and we can do that knowing Poppa is now safe and sound.

Thank all of you for being there and we will be in contact.

Later, David

* * * * *

Dear Cyber Friends gathered about me,

Just to let you know that at 3:26 this afternoon Poppa took his last deep breath, let it out and headed back to The Stars, into the arms of the Lord and the Bosom of Abraham, back from whence he came, back to Mother Spider, quit this life. It was deeply peaceful and gracious, a teacher even to his last breath.

We're both now very tired, greatly relieved and quite all right. Until later. Thanks for being there. Rebecca

E-mail of the day

Dear Ones,

I'm glad the end was so peaceful and now you both can rest. You'd probably sleep for a week if you could, and the grief brings it's own exhaustion. It's a perfect time of year to cozy up after the final arrangements, and hibernate. What sort of final memorial are you planning...did you plan with him?

I just have to say, Reb, that your letters have been wonderful to read...you write so beautifully and expressively that it's been a pleasure to read them.

My thoughts are with you still in this time, for it's not over til you're finished dealing with the memorial and relatives, there may still be trials to face. Take care. Love....RR

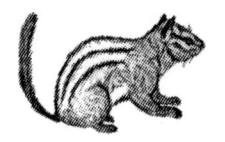

Lessons

Dying to learn

> *"...The conquest of the fear of death is the recovery of life's joy...the conquest of the fear of death yields the courage for life."*
> Joseph Campbell, *The Power of Myth*

About my parents.

Perhaps, dear Reader, you have wondered at the titles I have given my parents. When I was twelve years old, my parents separated me from my brothers, and took me into the dining room to tell me that I had been adopted by them at the end of The War. Thirty years later, on my last visit with my mother, when I was an adult and a mother myself, I queried her about my adoption. Probably without thinking she mentioned something about my having known my father until I was seven years old, the year our family moved to London. When I asked her what he had been like, she grew agitated and muttered: "It's all so long ago, I don't remember!" Then she had thrust a mildewed book at me. It was the handbook for adopting war orphaned children published by His Majesty's Stationers.

There was a section on how adopting parents were to tell the child of its heritage. My parents had followed that lesson to the letter.

When I first heard the news that I was adopted, I felt as if the carpet had been pulled out from under my feet, and I found not a sturdy, steady floor beneath, only a vacant sky. From that date until after I left my mother's home, I had a recurring nightmare of being smothered by a roiling greyness. That I was adopted made a lot of sense for it explained so much, that gender did not, about how differently from the brothers of my childhood, I looked at life.

One of the complaints the mother of my childhood would lob at me during our tension-filled years together was that I was far too selfish, far too self-absorbed. Now I know that that is one of the wounds an adopted child unwittingly carries around. For adoption is a genetic amputation leaving ghostly feelings of separateness, unconnectedness. Perhaps more than anybody else, we adopted children are beset with an invisible heritage from which we cannot draw any frames of reference as to who we are, where we come from, how we fit in and where we will be going.

When I reached my majority, she ordered me to stop calling her any name denoting mother. When I asked in exasperation, what I should call her, she fired back that she'd rather I didn't call her anything. Thus, she became the mother of my childhood. The last time I wrote to her, some twenty years later, was my 'thank-you letter' and in it I addressed her by her first name and surname. Whether she wanted to read it or not, I closed that letter with my love and thanks for having given me a good start in life.

Wondering about death.

As a child, Life came and went by me; the seasons turned; our family ate meat and I never thought about what had had to die that we might eat; we grew and harvested vegetables from our garden and plucked fruit from the orchard. It was all there for us. Life simply went on, seemingly seamlessly and endlessly.

Then we moved to London and I was old enough to begin understanding The War stories that abounded in every family's history. I listened to the memories of uncles and sons, husbands, brothers and fathers who never came home and I'd wonder why. Occasionally there was a hushed conversation in the sitting room from which I would be banished. One day, the King died and school was let out early. As I ran home, the grown-ups I passed sternly ordered me to walk. For months everything was in a grim, grey sadness as the nation mourned. Once a classmate's father died and she was absent for a week. Then Jo Hyde-Smith's husband Sam died, and I couldn't go play with their children for a while, and when we met again, no one talked about it.

Death swam into my ken when I was introduced to the historical plays of The Bard, *Macbeth*, *Hamlet*, *Henry V* and *Richard III*. During history classes I would notice the dates of the monarchs' reigns. Yet they were merely dusty dates, signifying nothing more than a part of a past about which we had to learn.

For some years in my teens, my mother dragged me to a Veterans' hospital where I was expected to read to a ward of wounded warriors. Left alone in a colorless dim room with a dozen beds in which blind and crippled men silently lay, I would pick up the day's newspaper and read out loud. The first time my mother dropped me off at the nurses' station, the ward nurse had instructed me not to talk to anyone in there, and so I spoke to no one and no one spoke to me. It was only after several weeks that I plucked up enough courage to say hello and identify myself when I entered, and to bid them all goodbye and tell them that I'd see them all again the next week. Only then did those sad and trapped men murmur replies. Occasionally, over the course of those years, I would arrive to find one of the beds empty. No one said anything.

Death, to adopted children, seems like something that happens all around us and, because we have no visceral connection other than our capacity for love and the comfort of familiarity, does not happen to us. Poppa's passing, for the first time in my life, gave me most of what I had missed, for I knew who I was, where I'd come from, how I fit in and where I was going.

Because of the way the family of my childhood coped with the death of its father, in hushed hidden conferences before I was exiled and in a rigid silence after I returned, I learnt to leave death to my elders.

My first funeral.

Standing The Watch is a phrase that has lingered in my psyche since my childhood. England then, was a society still steeped in the tradition of Standing The Watch as our monarchs died. I was too young for Queen Elizabeth's father's death to make much of an impression, other than to notice a general national somberness. It was when we all waited for Sir Winston Churchill to die, that I first truly had the experience of Standing The Watch. In my semi-classical education while England was in the death-throes of its empire, there were many famous paintings of dying kings and children, poets and knights. Those last thirteen days of Poppa's life felt like Standing The Watch.

I elicited a reaction of disbelief from my mother when, as an obedient daughter, I told her I was going to stand in line to pay my respects at the Lying in State of Sir Winston Churchill, a mighty presence in my childhood, whose voice and words had been indelibly imprinted on my psyche. I waited in the grey day, shuffling forward until I was inside the cathedral and followed the orderly queue toward the catafalque. It was there as I was absorbing the scene and saying my thanks, that the line of mourners halted as the ceremony of Changing the Honor Guard took place. Then, on the other side of the flag-draped bier, three heavily veiled women emerged from the shadows and the world stood still as The Queen, her mother and her sister paid their respects.

No one at home wanted to know about that. No one in my family to this day wants to talk about the death of our father, forty odd years past nor the death of our mother, just a decade ago. Writing this book has been the breaking of a huge taboo from my past. I have both hated and relished the process.

Of doctors and pastors.

You may have noticed that in this book doctors and pastors don't come off in a good light. I expect I will mightily offend those who believe in the powers of doctors and the righteousness of those who administer to our spiritual needs.

All my life I have been a patient patient, noticing how doctors talk to me about my health. In my work I have met many physicians of various healing persuasions, and I have found them all to be quite human with all the blind spots to which we are all heir. A thoracic surgeon probably knows as little about bunions and poison ivy as a pediatrician knows about geriatrics. A general practitioner understands less about female problems than his nursing assistant.

When we first came to this land, the doctor assigned to Poppa ran a practice that ranged from the cradle to the grave. When he knew he didn't know enough, he knew enough to confer with specialists. His successor was hired to focus on the cradle. Anyone wishing to grow old and die needed to go elsewhere. Because of our lifestyle and the health plan covering Poppa, we could not pick and choose.

With regard to my antipathy to holy men, I admit a prejudice. As someone who has read religious history and noted the misogyny, brainwashing and spiritual plunder therein, I hold no reverence for the henchmen of monotheism (the belief or doctrine that there is only one, masculine god.) Had I met Poppa during his missionary heyday, I would have beaten a rapid retreat, for I have no fondness for preachers of any bent. I have even less affection for hypocrites hiding behind mild-mannered, mealy-mouthed, fear-drenched scripts for as the shepherd teaches his flock, so shall his flock learn.

As my husband waded against the tide of current social customs to honor his vow to his father, I followed in his wake and observed the floundering of people who called themselves religious, watched their discomfort and fear when confronted with the unscripted experience of a home death.

Why a home death?

By all accounts, we had an easy home death. It didn't last long. There were no grim extended ailments and no devastating mental collapse. Poppa was a simple man, who died simply.

Why should anyone in their right mind think to give their loved-one a home death?

After all, our society is set up to take care of all of this dreadful business. We have nursing homes, hospitals, long-term care facilities, private elder care institutions, even hospices where those in the last sentences of their lives may be warehoused and cared for. All that is needed is money to buy such care. We didn't have that money, and I suspect millions of us don't.

Putting money aside, why else would adult children choose to bring their parents home to die? Somehow we modern children have decided that our parents aren't worth it. That we can't do it. We've been told often enough, to leave it all to those in the business. We'd just get in the way. We're not skilled enough to be in service to a home death. Just how many people do die at home these days?

I see ads on TV with elderly actors speaking seemingly thoughtful and kind lines about how they want to leave their children with an inheritance rather than debts, how they don't want to be a burden to their children. The idea that a person's dying is a burden, curdles my blood.

I suppose for a society that has only recently accepted the idea of a leave of absence for its workers when their offspring are born, the idea of another vacation, in order to bid their elders *bon voyage*, is a bit steep. Just as we think to hire strangers in strange places to help us with our births, we think of dying as a life's event we prefer not to face, and so we leave our elders to face it alone.

Don't get me wrong! A home death was no walk in a monastery of peace and harmony. We sweated anxiety when doses didn't work. We faced down ardent salesmen ever urging us on to bigger and better trappings for burials. We listened to the whining of a wimp of a pastor and the eager-beaver EMTs explaining just how they'd handle this cardiac patient, once they'd got their hands on him. The stuff of our days and nights was filled with ringing bells; wet sheets and overturned containers; of anguish and resistance.

Sometimes the alarm went off and we'd stumble along the damp, cool path only to find an old man sawing *zzzzs* like the venerable feller he was, while his gnarled hand gripped the bed rack at the exact spot of his alarm button.

There was anguish galore when scribbled instructions couldn't be deciphered, or when we had to call the home health nurses because we didn't know what was happening.

Certainly, annoyance would slice through the numbness of sleep deprivation, when the urine bag that I had to clean, slipped from my fingers and added yet another task, mopping the floor.

Slow and stead, make every step count, stay focused.

Frustration seethed when we waited for the doctor to write his scripts for necessities and medicines for Poppa's ease. *What part of pain did he not understand?*

Or, the despair when we had to tell this missionary of forty years in the fields of his Lord, that his pastor would not, could not come out to have one last prayer meeting with him.

Or, when that first home health nurse sat us down and asked us what our plans were. "I mean about after he dies, what are you going to do?"

While we may have been waiting for Poppa to die, there were huge lessons to be learnt. The waiting for returned phone calls seemed interminable. Especially when we realized: there was no waiting. We had to make every second count. That this was it!

That being said, a dying at home is a grand lesson in living in the here and now.

Step forward and breathe!

While a home death can be frightening, time-consuming, worrying, stressful, unpleasant and tiresome, it is also a fertile ground for courage, discipline, stamina, spirituality, compassion, loyalty, humor and love.

Why parents hide children from death.

Most modern parents want to shield their children from the horrible things in life, so why expose them to Death? I hope some of my story explains why. Keeping children away from the completion of a life, is to teach them only half of the equation. It keeps them in the dark, and cripples them emotionally and spiritually with a self-serving kind of protection that prevents children from wondering about why they are alive; blunts them from exploring the full range of their feelings.

We all live only to die. As winter dies so that spring can be born, summer dies so that autumn can come. For untold generations, children have been at the dying of relatives. It is only in this strange modern world that we hide them from such events, all the while encouraging them to save the world's climate, feed the world's hungriest and donate to the world's poorest. Meanwhile we inundate them with programs, films and games that mete out death by deletion, while giving them no insights as to what dying does to a body.

I know now that death is almost contagious. For a while there I was infected with a loss of impetus, a loss of purpose. *If this is what's in store, what is the point of all that I do every day?* For a week after Poppa's bag of bones was zipped into the body bag and driven off, I simply had no energy to do anything. It is a given that I was tired, yet there was something more—it wasn't exactly that I too wanted to die, it was more a feeling of what was the point all of this busy-ness? Grieving and depression were not in my family's vocabulary.

When I was exiled from my father's dying, there had been no one I could talk with about my feelings and questions. What did it all mean? Why am I feeling so useless? Where does Daddy go when he dies? Why can't I help? What happens to Daddy's body? Why am I so lethargic? What will happen to us all now? Why am I so sad all the time and cry at the slightest thing?

What have I learnt about dying.

When Brother Death comes to visit, our welcome is fraught with fear. Fear of the unknown both of what is to come and where our loved-one will be going.

When I set off from the London train station on my emigration, my loved-ones had no understanding of where I was going. I was taking the trip on pure faith that the train would safely arrive on the coast, and that the ship I was to take, would safely cross the Atlantic, cruise around the Statue of Liberty, and deposit me safely in the New World. Once landed, I would be safely on my way to America's heartland.

When Death is the next stop on our Cosmic Journey, we have to take it all on faith. That our service to the travelers, is all we have to offer. That those travelers are on their paths and rightly headed on their Way. Just as we linger after our loved-ones have gotten married and sped off on their honeymoon, we linger after death, to tidy up.

What about those urgings my husband and I were given that we should have Poppa committed to a home, where he could be taken care of properly? Our pledge to our beloved Poppa took care of that worry.

What about readjusting our lives so we could take care of our elder in the manner he deserved and requested? Being hired to care for this senior citizen allowed us to change our lifestyle so we could cater to his home death. All our needs were taken care of, even if our wants nagged at us now and again. It would have been nice if we could have traveled here, done this, bought that.

In a special little book, *The Third Eye*, which I had read during a particularly frightening period when I was new to motherhood, and trying to find a safe nest, there was a scene in which an elder quietly died, attended by a doctor and an acolyte from a nearby Tibetan lamasery. The memory of that scene surfaced frequently during Poppa's last days here on earth, and without that book, I would not have seen the Glow.

The costs of a home death.

I know that most of the costs of Poppa's dying at home were picked up by Uncle Sam, under the senior citizen just rewards system, petty bureaucracy notwithstanding. The wheels of that vast accounting house grind everso slowly, and for more than a year after his death, we were still receiving notifications of payments for this and for that. As Poppa had not been a Veteran, disposing of his earthly remains was left up to us.

A home death is quite economical. The State paid David an hourly wage for his caregiving, which was a quarter of all the wages and overheads professional institutions rack up and charge to the system, to us, the taxpayers.

I know we were fortunate that we could arrange our lives so we could honor our elder's wishes, and provide him with the exit of his choice. After all these years, I honor my mother for giving her husband the death of his choice, by keeping him home rather than washing her hands of the whole thing and shipping him off to a hospital, which had been her first reaction when she learnt he was in a terminal state.

As I served my husband's father in his needs during his final days, I was both stretched to my limits and yet invigorated. I was absorbed in each moment, and intensely aware of being alive. Should I have been tearing out my hair, wailing with grief? Perhaps when it is my husband's time, I'll experience such sorrow. I know when I contemplate the deaths of my children, a massive stunning ache accosts me.

What about grief?

As Poppa aged through his 80s, it was obvious his hourglass was almost full. Perhaps I am an oddity, because I felt no sorrow at the ending of a fully lived, long life. The sorrow came later, in spring when the bulbs bloomed and when David and I planted seeds. When we tended the garden, and ate of its bounty, and Poppa was not there to harvest and enjoy it.

I have known many people who carry grief around for not having made or taken the time to tell their loved-ones of their affection. In the aftermath of September 11, I have heard many say how glad they were to have told those who never came home that they were loved. It has been my practice to tell the people I love that I love them. For that I have no regrets, because I was with Poppa day and night, and told him, often, how much he meant to me.

Where we live, the nearest long-term facility is over an hour's drive away and, more like as not, Poppa would have been warehoused even further afield. This would have shifted our lives into a pattern of hurried, occasional visits to an impersonal place in which Poppa had no anchor, memories nor frames of reference. Those places rarely have sleeping-in facilities for visiting family, so our lives would have become a desperate shuffle of our time, and a breeding ground for resentment as we attempted to do our duty by our elder. This home death eliminated all of that.

Talking about people who have died.

Poppa belonged only to my present. We had no mutual past other than the one we had made together in those last few years. Whatever sense of burden or annoyance at who he was and how he lived, sloughed away during the weeks we were finding out about his health.

To this day, David and I often reminisce about his presence in our lives. Perhaps a blue jay will squawk at us as we put out feed, or a chipmunk will scamper across the picnic table as I sit there writing, and Poppa will spring to mind. Perhaps one of us will remember one of his stories and recount it. Or when I am over in Poppa's cabin, I'll glance up at the photo of him and his wife that we still have hanging on a wall, and a moment in our lives together will flood my mind. Perhaps David will come across a tool from his father's ancient store, and he'll remember where and when they had first used it.

I have listened to the way people talk about someone who had just died. We still think of dying as a failure, just as we still think of the team that made the least goals, as losers. We haven't gotten to the way of thinking that without that team, there would be no winners. We still don't talk about how a good game was played by all. Obviously, someone has to lose, and just as obviously one team has to win. How we played the game is much more important, isn't it?

I know that Poppa's dying was the natural course of things, and we had the time to get used to it. We had little catching up to the idea. When people die before their time, so to speak, other emotions are tapped into—rage and impotence. I cannot speak to how I would feel then, except to think that we have to catch up, after the fact, to the idea of our loved-one's death. We have to get used to a future that would not now happen; accept all the loving memories that would not now be made.

Of passion and play.

I have been told I needed to put more passion into writing about the hours and days of our Standing The Watch. Most of my passion was spent by the time David and Poppa returned from Seattle, and I learnt how long Poppa had left. Instantly there bloomed within me a great relief, as well as a resolve to see it through, to honor my word.

It is my children who have shared my passions, for they were the ones who gave me my connection to humanity. That connection was both shocking and exhilarating. It was as if I had discovered a string of Christmas lights, slid the plug into a socket and *voilá*, excitement, memory, feelings, and a deep visceral jolt into the world of family. After my daughter was born, I felt, for the first time, another's pain and wonder, fear and courage, anger and love, sorrow and satisfaction, and in doing so, learnt what parts of my emotional rainbow had been dimmed by lack of kin.

As my emotions reconnected, I uncovered a horde of not-so-happy memories of a girlhood among boys, among other girls, and among Christian aristocrats. The body remembers, even when the mind wills amnesia. The tsunami of motherhood washed over me, as I became aware of being genetically, kinetically reconnected with another human. My arid emotional landscape became saturated with the milk of human kindness, and produced an abundance of intense, immense emotions, clear across the spectrum. Once upon a time my children were the only reason I kept going. They were the sunshine that could brighten any drab day.

Poppa and I liked each other well enough, yet our relationship was always one of work. Poppa didn't know how to play. If he was not working, he was sleeping. Play was a sinful waste of time. He did not, as did my family and the family I made with my children, hold useful, games of any sort: not of playing cards, learning to read, figuring and writing, nor of strategy and memory.

    The playing of games was a big part of getting to know people, when I came up in those pre-television city times. We played games in our spare time, after our homework was done and when it was raining outside, when cousins came together, and during birthday parties. Playing games taught us how we felt about losing, what it was like to win, and how to play a good game. Games taught us about rules and goals in a gladsome way, which gave us practice in following, leading, being part of a team and being on one's own in a group, where all were determined not to lose. We even played a card game called Cheat! which encouraged us to break the rules. Games gave us a finite and safe space to practice our passions in losing without rancor or seeking revenge, and winning without arrogance. For without losers, there would be no winners. As a mother teaching her children how to play games, I also learnt how to assist them in winning, for as an adult, always winning over my children was no fun! Always, I asked if they'd enjoyed playing the game; if it had been a good game, no matter who won.

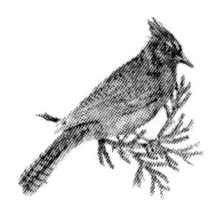

How then will we die?

Another sunrise

*"...to say we end
The heart-ache and the thousand natural shocks
That flesh is heir to..."*
      William Shakespeare, *Hamlet, Prince of Denmark*

Sit with me, dear Reader, a while longer in another sunrise.

As a child, born of the energy of war, among a people who had collectively known death by unnatural causes, twice in their lifetime, I frequently heard my elders speak some variation of: "Wouldn't you rather die of old age at home in your bed?" Often uttered as a *"...consummation devoutly to be wish'd."*

While the revered Bard's plays rarely included characters going through that most authentic of experiences, his emphasis lay after all, in our passion for being alive, he did allow a couple of old warriors such a death. Mostly, though, the dialogue moaned about the despair of growing old, not of the adventure of dying.

Growing old is not for the faint of heart. Over the years, as I watched Poppa slowly make his way from this world, I experienced the full spectrum of those emotions to which we are heir.

Most of us easily identify six basic emotions: Fear, Anger, Hate, Grief, Love and Contentment. We get confused when joy is blended with grief, when depression follows bliss. Getting hurt emotionally, comes from other people's way of treating us. Thus we think of our emotions as involuntary reactions, rather than practiced responses. While we ache to express ourselves spontaneously, we must survive years of training in how to handle our emotions. Even so, we let people push our buttons rather than learn to play with our feelings, which we think of as unruly aberrations, rather than guides to living in a state of consciousness.

Like people who live near the North Pole who have many names for snow, or people who live with rain who have many ways to describe all the different kinds of downpours, we, of the temperate zone, have many ways to explain our emotions. English is a language filled with euphemisms, hyperbole and similes.

Fear: disquiet, uneasiness, dread, apprehension, trepidation, worry, discomposure.

Hate: resentment, malice, contempt, animosity, jealousy, envy, greed, hostility, revenge.

Anger: outrage, fury, shame, pride, temper, indignation, displeasure, impatience, annoyance, violence, tantrum, petulance, conniption, bile.

Grief: remorse, sorrow, sadness, melancholy, despondency, anguish, misery, despair, depression.

Love: passion, infatuation, sensuality, lust, desire, rapture, ecstasy, elation, warmth, affection, sympathy, empathy, tenderness, concern, pathos, bathos.

Contentment: satisfaction, happiness, delight, glee, thrill, bliss, elation, inspiration.

During those last thirteen days of my father-in-law's life, I experienced every one of those emotions. They would gush up like a blush. I did nothing about them, simply observed them, and lived through to the other side. After all, Standing The Watch wasn't about me.

Did you notice that Reverence was not in that list?

As an art student in my teens, I saw many *Pietas*, those statues of a cloaked woman holding a naked dying man. In discussing those works of art, my teachers avoided mentioning death, as if it was a given. Rather they focused on the skills of the artists, and how the statues evoked emotions. What I saw was something eternal and deeply affecting. Those statues are much more than Christian imagery, they are a universal expression of reverence. As an early Feminist, I often reversed the genders: imagined a cloaked man holding a near-naked dying woman. Changes one's perspective a bit.

I realize that in today's climate, revering our elders is politically incorrect. Instead we are expected to worry more about the living conditions of our prisoners, and the morals of our politicians.

Meanwhile here in America, more people are maturing into eldership than ever before. Soon, no matter our ethnic roots, our age will make us a majority.

So how then will we die?

If we do not practice reverence for our elders, how then will we be treated when we mature, and our time comes?

There's something about caring for our parents in their last days that is more spiritual than all the religious words any holy man could say. More rewarding than any other work ethic. Somehow we've gotten the idea that we're not religious enough to Stand The Watch, that dying like being born, is an event best ministered to by professionals.

When I was in service to Poppa on his way back to the stars, anger and fear, grief and joy, pathos and bathos rippled through me like waves on a lake after a trout has flown for a fly.

Anger is an old combatant of mine. It has had me by the short hairs a time or two, especially when confronted with social injustice or personal disrespect. The anger I felt during Poppa's dying, was only toward the way bureaucracies grind a person down, no matter on which side of the counter we stand, until there is only the begging.

The anger I felt at the clergy in Poppa's life was undoubtedly mixed with contempt for one particular fainthearted fellow. And last, although certainly not the least, was the anger I felt for the doctor assigned to Poppa in his final years. That anger curdled into rage when I realized he knew about as much as I did, and then did a disappearing act when the going got tough.

Fear, I have also known from early years. As the only girl in a bunch of older boys; my first nights away at boarding school; being surrounded by a racist mob; seeing evil intent in a person's face; walking into a dangerous moment in other people's homes.

During my walk through the Valley of Death, I felt fear for how little I knew about dying. Like everyone else, I have visions of Death draped in dreadful robes, carrying a sweeping scythe. That image is far older than those bright scenes of a jovial, eternal Santa Claus, or a bouncing beautiful New Year Babe. It is a conscious effort for me to balance the dark with the light. Luckily I have an everyday example of when night gives way to day.

Hate too, has dogged my footsteps. Sometimes I didn't know why it was directed at me, and sometimes I did. When I was young, I relished hating things, people and places. I hated my heavy glasses that brought insults down on me; the gap between my front teeth that gave me a lisp; my Scripture Class teacher for humiliating me; my brothers' teasing that got me into trouble; school bullies who trapped me into fights; tripe and onions which nauseated me; and cold, dank bed sheets.

I loathed math because I couldn't wrap my mind around its abstractness. Oh, I could count, multiply, subtract and divide. Anything more confounded me, and I hated that confusion.

As I grew up, I hated the way my elders thought the worst of me, and the way men talked down to me, simply because of my gender. It was the feeling of hate that finally drove me out of the country of my childhood to a land where I thought I could leave all that hate behind: the hatred of strangers, of different kinds of people, of religions, accents, social expectations and classes. *Out of the frying pan, into the fire!*

The hate I felt during Poppa's dying was about doing things like wiping up runny feces or vomit, spilled urine or food. The hate would rush through me like a flash flood, leaving behind a field of relief; and I would simply finished the task.

Grief comes to us all: for small things like a wounded pet, the loss of a job, the breaking of a favored treasure, as well as for huge things like a besmirched planet, a lost love, an untimely end to a life, a dream, a hope. Grief seeps into our hearts as surely as plaque into our veins; stiffening our emotions until they are brittle; saturating our feelings with gloom.

Grief teaches us that even as we weep for what is lost, we must take that next breath. Grief is a many-textured emotion that comes upon us like a dark cloud, shutting out the light, dimming our delights and wrapping us up in sorrow. Grief, as with all emotions, is simply to be experienced, lived through, and when the misery rinses out of our system, contentment will replenish us.

Contentment. Perhaps of all the emotions, contentment, for wherein I find myself, has been my daily manna and mantra. The feeling of rightness in what I was doing in the service to this elder and his son, nourished me as only the milk of human kindness can.

*　　　*　　　*　　　*　　　*

While dying comes to us all, all of us do not come to dying easily. We have old saws that remind us to live each day, as if there is no tomorrow; we speak new aphorisms about telling our loved-ones of our love, as if they will not return to us. We take seminars on how to give of our love so it will grow, rather than hoarding it away for some unspecified rainy day. As if we have as finite a quantity of emotions, as we do days.

I am not urging you, dear Reader, to put your house in order and sit back and wait for your death. I am, however, encouraging you to consider how you would like your parents' dying to be and by extension, yours and your children's.

For most of us, discarding all our worldly belongings and flying off to work among the destitute and dying, is not an option. For most of us, taking care of our parents as they die, is.

Did your parents abandon you as a child, leave you to raise yourself alone? Or did they devote decades of their lives to nurture you to maturity? Yes, I'm sure, in the beginning it was as a result of that old black magic called Biology, when spring sprang in their loins and the world was all a-twitter with lust, romance and the survival of the species. Later, as you became a family member, it was from their own motives of love and pride and satisfaction.

Now your parents are on their way to their next adventure, and you are left wondering about this thing called Death. Standing The Watch at a home death offers an experience as authentic as a home birth. Even if it is impossible to bring your parents home, consider devoting your life for the duration of their dying. I'm not referring to a long convalescence or an interminable age-related deterioration (although many of us will step forward in service to those), I'm simply speaking of the days of dying. When everyone knows the end is nigh. When all that is left is the leaving. When the bag of bones is being vacated as the Spirit readies to soar aloft.

Whichever way of Standing The Watch for your loved-ones you choose, you will not be alone. There are all sorts of people, in all sorts of spiritual expressions who can walk through the Valley of Death with you. There is also a myriad of people in social agencies who must accompany you. You get to choose many of them, just as you choose who will be at the birth of your children. And just as in a home birth, a home death is not about you or the people in its service, it is about those who are doing the dying. So, don't let the professionals make you cower!

I keep coming back to the birth process. Once it is over with, most of us forget about the negatives and remember the awe, the thrill, the bliss. For unto you your child was born. Even to this day, with my kids full grown, I seldom remember the bad, and clearly see the good times.

I want to tell you that all the questions I had during this home death vanished in those last days; how they were no longer of any importance, because now I knew.

All the emotions vanished at the moment of death. Any grief was soothed by the contentment and satisfaction of a service well done; a good death was had. Because I was there all of the time, any disquiet or unease dissolved during the days of dying, for I had worked through them.

In Standing The Watch you will find much to be grateful for; you will be able to bask in your memories; sift through the bad and the good, until they are all rinsed clean by compassion and affection. For underlying your commitment to Standing The Watch, is your wonderment at how you, in time, will be remembered.

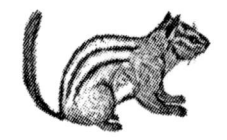

Connections

And life goes on

Dear Cyber friends,

Thank you for your comforting emails and for reminding me how life rolls right on. We're going through periods of relief and busy-ness, and then a sudden seeping away of energy, a dense sense of gravity, and all we can think to do is lay back in our recliners and sleep.

Buddy-dog is also slow and low and very clingy, confused to be all alone in the back seat of the minivan, when we drove out to Port Angeles yesterday, to take care of cremation and cemetery details. It was a hard, long day that started before dawn, and ended when we rolled back in the dark and rain to a cold cabin. The glass-door wood stove, Brother Michael gave us, heats our little home quickly and soon we were dozing before the TV, also a gift from that Spirit Brother.

Poppa had reiterated his wishes to us several times: no funeral, no services and no flowers. If anyone wanted to make a Memorial Gift in his name, he asked that they endow their church Missionary Fund.

While going through Poppa's wallet, we came upon $23 and in celebration, while we were in Port Angeles, we took a rest at the Golden Gate, eating our favorite dinners and toasting Poppa with our tea and soda. It was a delicious meal and the waitress, Mary, who knows us well from the decade we've been eating there, brought three fortune cookies, as she always did. Poppa's was already cracked and said: *Your work is done.*

How are we doing? We're plodding. I figure we're both in the Shock stage of Grieving. I've been over in Poppa's cabin, a morning habit and ritual I find comforting, to clean and tidy and be in his presence. I've been cutting up his pajamas to make a quilt for the guest bed. Took out my sewing machine, as well as the keyboard Michael gave me for my birthday, which I play now and again. My beloved is absorbed in reading and working on his computer. We talk and talk, he of his memories of his father and me of my feelings.

For much of September and all of October, I've lived with a knot in my gut and an adrenaline squirt every few hours as Poppa's failing systems brought about dramatic episodes. For weeks we've lived on twelve hour shifts. As David would come to bed in the predawn hours, I would rise and begin the trips over to Poppa's side to ease the pain, cleanse and comfort. He did enjoy having his back swabbed with rubbing alcohol and then blown upon, cooled him off.

For those final thirteen days, from the Wednesday in Seattle when Poppa and David received the surgeon's death sentence, until the day, out here in the wilderness, when Poppa took his last breath, we did double duty because we both needed the support. To the end Poppa took care of us. Perhaps he knew our systems wouldn't have been able to keep it up much longer. Now we're allowing ourselves to rest, work a little like hauling in wood, changing out water, answering e-mails and then napping again. Once a day, come rain or dry, we walk to the bridge and back, retracing Poppa's daily trek and seeing it now in all its sodden autumnal splendor!

Great is the gap this Old Soul has left. We're fine with it all, just tired. Pondering on life and dying, funerals and pastors, rip-off oil-and-lube companies and other earthly matters!

I was packing things away for Goodwill, listening to Poppa's TV, when I smelt an awful burning, and Lo, if the picture didn't distort like taffy and die.

I find myself often singing this hymn.

> *Now I walk in beauty*
> *Beauty is before me*
> *Beauty is behind me, above and below me.*

as well as:

> *I will be gentle with myself*
> *I will love myself*
> *I am a child of the Universe*
> *Being born each moment.*

I'll say goodbye for now. I thank you for your comforting connection and you know I love you, Rebecca

E-mails of the day

> Rebecca, you can always make me cry...in the best way. Your story helps me hold my Dad closer, even though he died in 1991. Love is where it's at, isn't it? Sorry to know that you lost your father

when you were so young, a hug for you, as always. Love, Lynn.

* * * * *

Dear Reb....Thought I'd check in on you. How are things going? Life is probably really different this winter and it's nice this is the deep quiet time to let the grief you must feel be as it needs to be before the rebirth of Spring.

In my experience Grief is in 3 stages:

1. Shock which lasts weeks and in which reality is very strange.

2. Settling In which is a tearful, erratic time of open grief lasting months, and

3. Status Quo the deep quiet grief of missing and feeling the empty, unfilled space left by the beloved, often lasting years.

Let me know how you are doing, I love the way you write as you are so wonderfully articulate.

Take care.... blessed be....RR

* * * * *

Dear Rebecca and Dave,

Talking with you and Dave has helped me an awful lot also. I have really not been healing the way I should. I miss my Papa more than anyone in the family except my mom.

We visit the graveyard at least twice a month but I have other siblings who weren't even interested in the arrangements at the time or even going to visit Papa now. That makes me a little sad, when I ask them about going they just tell me, "Who wants to go see some dead guy's grave?" It was the same with the arrangements also no one except my youngest sister, who couldn't afford it either, was the one who helped the most. I guess it is that way in every family.

You may keep that Hospice paper I made that copy for you and Dave, I am sorry it came late, maybe at a time you can pass it along to someone else in need.

I am happy and your Poppa would be also that you had a supper toasting him, so true to life sometimes are the fortune cookies...and they don't even know it.

Mom is doing very well, she has an ulcer on her leg but I am doctoring it for her and making her booboo much better...if only she minds and keeps her feet up.

Well, dear friend of the e-Mail and my happier childhood home, I will say so long for now but if you and Dave need anything please feel free to write or call.

Make yourself happy and you can make people around you happy.

I love the songs you sent,
Love to you and Dave also, May

*   *   *   *   *

Dear Rebecca,

As always it is good to hear from you, I have been thinking about you a lot. Wanting to give you space to adjust and be.

Thanks for your kind words, I learned a tremendous amount from your sharing, it meant so much to me—you are such an inspiration. I applaud all the years you took care of Lincoln and how you were there for him in death. I am glad to hear that all is well, I knew once you started getting some rest, things would start looking up.

I remember the first Thanksgiving you and David were together in Sequim, I drove with the kids through the snow, I remember the roads were hairy, the food great and the company great. And I remember a Thanksgiving before that, celebrated with you, Bati and Ben, William, Cam and Beth here around the table in the sun room. I have a great photo of it, the kids look so young!

I would love to have you both, you can always retreat to the cabin, we will bring turkey over! I still do want to visit you.

Love, love and love, Deborah

* * * * *

Reb,

God bless Poppa and you two. You did a wonderful job helping Poppa exit this existence. You will be blessed. Faina.

* * * * *

Reb, I'm so grateful that Poppa went peacefully and gracefully and could be at home with you, David and Buddy. I can imagine your relief and extreme exhaustion. Now, you rest my friends. Love, Jane

* * * * *

Good morning David and Rebecca,

Aunt Betty called us last evening with the news that Uncle Lincoln had died. I had planned to send him a newsy E-mail today just to say I loved him and share some memories. Couldn't do that so I just spent some time "talking to him." Then I got to thinking of he, Daddy and Aunt Mabel in heaven all together. What a gathering!

I have such fond memories of Uncle Lincoln and they will always remain in a special place in my heart. He was a dear special, tough and yet tender man. Those of us who had the privilege of knowing and loving him were indeed lucky.

Thank you for the special care you both gave him these many years. We shall be praying for you both as you take care of the many details involved at this time. Just know that God is looking upon you with a smile and a grateful heart for having loved Uncle Lincoln so much.

Love, Karen

*   *   *   *   *

David,

My sis Karen called and said Linc had died. Reminded me of a story he told me quite some time back.

Apparently he and Eva were driving somewhere in the southwest and he came up a rise and heard the choir of angels singing. Linc described it as the most beautiful music he had ever heard. And he was looking forward to hearing it again.

I believe that is happening now. And to those of his family left, remember he is only finishing the trip he started a long time ago. Also he is in a better place to intercede for us when we make that same journey.
  Love to all
  Clyde & Sylvia

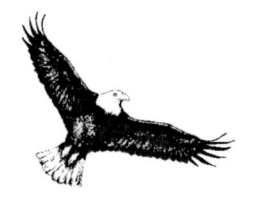

Another gift from the Cosmos

> *"Today as in ancient times, collective rituals that re-create the origins of the world renew the community by reconnecting people with the rhythmic source of their being. Our rituals function as a gateway...into deeper realms of consciousness. The rhythms of our drums have the power to draw listeners away from the constraints of clock time back to the cyclical time of mythology."*
> Layne Redmond, *When the Drummers Were Women*

The Cosmos gave me a second chance with David's father and I was deeply honored to have been in service to this fine Old Soul as he crossed over The Veil and the Father of my childhood was very close at that time, for Poppa had become my own father.

Unlike my father, who was given a well-scripted funeral service performed by the holy men of his faith and a somber midwinter burial, attended by family, business colleagues, and the men of his religious community, Lincoln Brown had wanted "no fuss, no muss." He had asked that there be no service presided over by a pastor, no relatives expending finances they could not afford to come in from afar and no graveside ceremony as his ashes were deposited. He had growled that as he wouldn't be there, he didn't care for all that fancy stuff.

With Michael John Barbee's dying, the Cosmos gave me the gift and opportunity to create a Ceremony of Celebration for someone I loved. With Percy, MerryJo and Lincoln enfolded in my heart, and in tandem with my husband, I set about Celebrating A Life.

Michael was our beloved Spirit Brother who came to stay with us over the New Year, a year after Poppa's Death. That visit turned out to be the last time we'd ever see him on this side of the Veil, for one Friday in January, while he was napping, his body had a massive cerebral hemorrhage and died. His father called us to ask that we come be with him. He was lost and didn't know what next to do.

At Father Bob's home we met up again with Michael's daughter who was now fifteen, the same age I had been when my own father had died.

After we'd all put the pieces together, we realized that for weeks Michael had been giving us clues. David and he had even had an earnest exchange about him going to the ER or a doctor, when he described symptoms of a stroke. This very private man said no, "can't be bothered with those quacks" This was his path, and he was following it.

When Amy handed me one of her father's tie-dyed T-shirts that I had so loved, warm from the dryer, I burst into tears and buried my face in it, as I had done just three weeks before when I had bid my Spirit Brother farewell. Michael's daughter extracted my promise that I would wear it with my blue jeans skirt and our Poppa's red suspenders at the Ceremony.

What a jangle of feelings is grief, immense moments when the seduction of dying sucks strong on the Spirit, almost as if fighting against dying has become an addiction, and we're so tired of wrestling against it. Why not simply concede and go with the flow?

Other moments, when friends drop by with dinner, a bouquet of carnations, a bag of jigsaw puzzles and bright encouragement, I remember how good it is to be alive. Far from the madding crowd might seem bliss to someone in a seething city. Coyotes, however, don't cook; cougars don't do dishes and trees are wooden when it comes to sorrow or ecstasy!

What is this hunger that has me eager for the next moment here on Earth? If life is so hard, why don't we have raucous Bon Voyage parties instead of weeping woeful wakes? If, where we're headed is so much better, why aren't we glad to be going? Whatever happened to the first three letters in the word funeral?

I used to think that it was better to be leaving than staying behind. In my early years, before boarding school, I'd pack for my brothers and see them off. Such a hullabaloo, off to see the World! Then it was my turn and the World was a lot scarier than I had expected! Not that my nest was that safe or welcoming, it was, however, familiar. Soon my boarding school became familiar and, at times, enjoyable, so much so that I came to dread returning home. Then I left the land of my childhood, of my maidenhood and my first years of work, for the New World and a new life. Decades later I was the one staying behind as my children left for their adult lives. And then I left the mainstream for a little eddy of land on the edge of civilization.

In contemplating my beloved Michael's death, a year after Poppa's and so sudden, so unexpected, I realized he could have died in any number of ways on his annual migration from the sodden Northwest winter, to the deserts of the Southwest, where he recharged his batteries with the energy of the communities he found there. As he meandered, he basked in the sun and the dryness, until he became a Terra Cotta Man. So whenever Michael headed out, I would say my goodbyes, and tell him I loved him as if I'd never see him again.

When he last left here, we hugged and kissed and bid farewell in our usual way, lingering with another story, another thought. All that I have now are the memories, just like everyone else who has ever had someone die. Knowing Brother Michael, I'd say he left exactly the way he wanted to, quietly heading out for his next adventure.

Brother Michael was a tease. You would hear him say, "Nanee-nanee-nanee!" He'd dance about, a bit like a boy with a secret, and you knew he'd just got one over on you. He was an explorer, with his eyes on the horizon and the sun at his shoulder. He loved to watch the life of the eagle families unfold in the copse across the fields from the home he so enjoyed. I would sometimes watch with him, for in that view I also saw beyond to the panorama of the Olympic Mountains in all their seasonal glory. Now Michael is soaring with his eagles.

Michael's father invited us out to eat after we'd been at his home, working on the Memorial Service, and tying up the loose ends of Michael's computer work, business world and generally giving his heir her due.

Michael's father had collected his son's ashes from the crematoria, and placed them on the passenger seat of his van as he drove home, admonishing his son not to comment on his driving. David asked Father Bob if Michael had nagged him, and the old man, who went to sea at the age of sixteen and plied merchant and supply ships all over the world during WWII, chuckled, "Not this time!" Then he showed us the elegant box in which Michael's ashes reposed, and we wept, hugging it to us, remembering all the times we had hugged his beloved bag of bones, and then we left Amy alone with her father.

When Amy joined us again, she said she wasn't hungry. Nonetheless, we repaired to Gwennie's and suddenly, when ordering, Amy's appetite returned, and she chose what she'd always eaten with her Dad, chicken strips and salad—ate ravenously too!

It was so good, the four of us sitting in that familiar restaurant, with the Sequim sun glowing. We asked Father Bob for stories from his past and he perked up, a flush came to his old face and he told us some fine yarns! Then, when David shared some of his stories and asked a question, Father Bob responded with a saying that Michael had also used, in just the same intonation and timbre, and it brought tears to our eyes and smiles to our lips. Father and son had the same hands and stance. Amazing is this genetic inheritance!

So, the Memorial was planned, and Amy wrote a moving poem. It was to be a full regalia Drum Circle which Michael so loved, and the funeral home would video tape the ceremony.

The next Saturday, we all arrived at the chapel in Port Angeles, and Smudged In in the bright winter sunshine. The funeral home dark-suited gentlemen looked confused and worried, as our motley crowd casually arrived with only the odd mourner in black. Everyone else was wearing their finest glad rags! In Michael's life on the Olympic Peninsula he had met and made friends with all sorts of folks, and we mingled together, some meeting each other for the first time: uncles, nephews, aunts and cousins; brothers, lovers, friends, colleagues and customers.

Michael's Ashes and his Buddha reposed on the Chapel Altar, along with flowers and cards from well wishers near and far. We moved the chapel chairs into semicircles around the Community Altar on which were set the Direction Candles, the Elements and the noisemakers.

Amy lit the Candles as she had done so many times at Drum Circles, and coherently spoke of her father, joining in the singing of familiar Circle songs. She had brought half a dozen of her school chums, most of whom got the giggles, which Michael would have enjoyed. He was ever one to giggle at seriousness! I could see the elders, invested in their serious sorrow, scowling at us youngsters, who just had no respect for the dead.

I had been gently beating a heartbeat on the great Heart Drum since the start, and when we got to the drumming, I felt Michael's energy swoop into me and he took us on a blood rushing gallop. That little chapel throbbed with so much life, I saw rainbows in the air!

There was much laughter and tears in the Telling of Michael. He was a tease and a trickster. He loved a good prank and royally pissed off a lot of folks. His brothers and his aunt told us of their joy with him. One brother spoke of how, while driving home to Seattle after helping his dad with Michael's stuff, a Red Hawk (one of Michael's Spirit Guides) had flown parallel to him all the way around Sequim Bay. One of his school chums spoke of the rock-'n'roll band they'd had together in their teens.

When George led us in The Om, the vibrations were ragged in the beginning as people got the hang of it. By the fourth intoning, it had become tight and harmonious, enfolding us in unity.

As we celebrated this bright Soul's Life, a group of his friends at the Tucson Gem Show (where Michael had rented a booth) was also drumming, as well as another group of friends near Cool, California. In Hawaii, Luke said he would be surfing and joining in the Bob Marley festival, and would raise a "cool one" to his Lodge Brother.

Then, when we had all spoken our names in Witness to this gathering, David uttered what Michael had always said as he left us: "Well, back to work!" And we all joined in laughing and that was it! Except for returning of the chapel to its former order, gathering up our playthings and our saying our farewells outside in the waning winter sunshine!

After letting Buddy-dog out for a relief run, David and I drove to The Golden Gate Restaurant with our Son who had come all the way from Seattle. Ben is a Lodge Brother, a member of a small group of men who used to come together in spiritual and spirited brotherhood, to initiate the young and tell the wise stories of the older men's lives about learning to walk their paths as Men.

There, after we had eaten, we talked with Ben about his wedding coming up in the Summer.

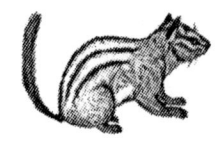

The Days of Lincoln Brown

1910-1999

Lincoln Brown went Home to the Lord
this 8th Day of November 1999
from his home in the Pacific Northwest.
He was born at home on August 6, 1910
on a sharecropped farm near Hallowell,
in Cherokee County, Kansas.
The eldest son of ten children
born to Abraham Lincoln Brown (b.1856)
and Bessie Brown (b.1880? née Davis).

Lincoln worked the farm and helped his mother raise the rest of their family after his father left. He had a natural ability for mathematics and all things mechanical, and earned his Journeyman Cards in several Trades including Carpentry, Machinery and Electrical. Lincoln worked at building and running of wood mills and smelting plants.

When Lincoln worked in the mines, he set the record for shoveling by hand the most ore in a single shift, and there once was a commemorative plaque for this feat in the Mining Museum in Joplin, Missouri.

Lincoln first came to the Olympic Peninsula in the 1930s to work in the lumber camps around Forks, along the Calawah and Bogachiel Rivers. During WWII his mechanical skills were in such high demand that he was recruited to maintain machinery for the war effort.

In 1947, while working along the Idaho/Washington border building grain silos, Lincoln was Saved and called to do the Work of the Lord. He also met and married his second wife, Eva Knickenbocker. They became Missionaries, traveling the Pacific Rim, the US and Alaska, as well as staying a few years in the Four Corners Reservations of the Southwest.

In 1980 Lincoln and Eva retired to the Sequim, Washington area where Eva went Home to the Lord six years later, and Lincoln moved in with their son, David.

Lincoln's greatest joy in his last years, was the telling of the stories of his life. He was also comforted and entertained by his doting companion, Buddy-dog. They were a fixture along the road, as they walked in all weather. His epitaph reads:

Here Lies A Good Man

A passel of comforting books

A One-Legged Cricket
by C. J. Macgenn
Publisher: iUniverse, Inc. 2001   ISBN: 0595168116
Subjects: 1) Psychology
         2) Allegory
         3) Love, Loss and Renewal

In this enchanting allegory, this author teaches us about grieving & loss, the depression & confusion after a loved-one's sudden death & how we can let go so that we may rebuild our lives. Reviewed on rebeccasreads.com

Another Country: Navigating the Emotional Terrain of Our Elders
by Mary Pipher, Ph.D.
Publisher: Riverhead Books 1999 ISBN: 1573221295
Subjects: 1) Aging parents–United State–Care.
         2) Adult children–Family relationships.
         3) Loss (Psychology) in old age.

A field guide to this foreign landscape of our parents as they grow older & we must talk with them about love & hygiene, loneliness, medicine, dependence & selling the car. Helpful in interpreting Poppa's frames of references, & what he had been going through in recent years. Reviewed on rebeccasreads.com.

Caregiver Therapy
by Julie Kuelbelbeck and Victoria O'Connor
Illustrations by R. W. Alley
Publisher: Abbey Press 1995   ISBN: 0870292854
Subjects: 1) Caregiving & Volunteers.
               2) Emotional Health.
               3) Aphorisms & hopeful ideas.
 Just the size to keep in your pocket to pull out during rough times. Kind & gentle sayings, with whimsical sketches, all designed to ease the stress of care givers. I used it often to catch my breath & validate where I was.

Deathing: An Intelligent Alternative for the Final Moments of Life
by Anya Foos-Graber
Publisher: Nicolas-Hays, Inc. 1989 ISBN: 0892540168
Subjects: 1) Spiritual Training
               2) Midwifing Dying
               3) The death moment
 Carolyn Stearns lent this to me, & it helped me remember what I felt & saw during Poppa's last thirteen days. It is a strange fascinatingly different way of thinking about how we can midwife dying & what happens to our Spirit, complete with exercises! A weird, satisfying read.

Do-It-Yourself Therapy: How To Think, Feel, and Act like a New Person In Just 8 Weeks
by Lynn Lott, Riki Intner and Barbara Mendenhall
Publisher: Career Press, Inc. 1999 ISBN: 1564144097
Subjects: 1) Psychological changes.
         2) Attitude changes.
         3) Personal consciousness.

You already know you can't change anyone else so here's help on how to change yourself; how to increase your self-awareness; transform your relationships & stop repeating self-defeating patterns. Really useful homework. Reviewed on rebeccasreads.com

Facing Death: Where Culture, Religion, & Medicine Meet
Edited by Howard M. Spiro, Mary G. McCrea Curnen and Lee Palmer Wandel
Publisher: Yale U. Press 1996   ISBN: 0300063490
Subjects: 1) Death–Psychological aspects.
         2) Moral, Religious, ethical aspects.
         3) Terminally ill.

This book helped turn us from viewing death as an adversary to accepting death as a defining part of life. A bit dry & academic, although very informative. Some really vivid passages of poems & pictures. Interesting morsels about death & dying from various religions.

Father-Loss: How Sons of All Ages Come to Terms with the Deaths of Their Dads
by Neil Chethik
Publisher: Hyperion 2001   ISBN: 0786865326
Subjects: 1) Psychology
          2) Loss and Bereavement
          3) Fathers and sons

I found this one during the writing of this book, & it opened up a whole new way of looking at my husband's grieving process. Men do grieve in difference ways from women. Reviewed on rebeccasreads.com.

Final Gifts: understanding the special awareness, needs, and communications of the dying
by Maggie Callanan and Patricia Kelley
Publisher: Bantam Books 1997   ISBN: 0553378767
Subjects: 1) Death–Psychological aspects.
          2) Terminally ill–Psychology.
          3) Terminally ill–Family relationships

Authentic stories of the special awareness, needs & communications of those nearing their dying & of their loved-ones. Kept us aware that others have been through this & what was happening for us all. Reviewed on rebeccasreads.com.

Final Passages: positive choices for the dying and their loved ones
   by Judith C. Ahronheim and Doron Weber
   Publisher: Simon & Schuster 1992   ISBN: 0671780255
   Subjects: 1) Death.
              2) Terminal care.
              3) Making choices.
A great comfort dealing with the terrors we had about Poppa's suffering & our facing Death. With chapters on Dying a Peaceful Death; How to Safeguard Your Legal Rights, & Expressing Your Feelings about Death. It was with us daily.

Finding the Way Home: a compassionate approach to illness
   by Gayle Heiss
   Publisher: QED Press 1997   ISBN: 0936609354
   Subjects: 1) Chronically ill–Family relationships.
              2) Healing–Psychological aspects.
              3) Helping behavior, Love, Grief, Death.
Based on the author's own experiences as well as hundreds of people who have attended her support groups, it explains the life-altering emotional & spiritual shifts when coming to terms with our dying. Changed our minds about the place of dying in the scheme of things.

Handbook for Mortals: guidance for people facing serious illness
by Joanne Lynn and Joan Harrold
Publisher: Oxford U. Press 1999   ISBN: 0195116623
Subjects: 1) Death.
2) Terminally ill.
3) Terminal care.

A warmly presented book for those who wish to approach their final years with a greater awareness of what to expect & greater confidence about how to make the end of our lives a time of growth, comfort & meaningful reflection. David found this one particularly comforting.

In the Arms of Others: a cultural history of the right-to-die in America
by Peter G. Filene
Publisher: I.R. Dee 1998   ISBN: 1566631882
Subjects: 1) Death.
2) Euthanasia–History–United States.
3) Medical technology.

This one takes us into the lives & feelings of people who have struggled with a modern dying. From the 19th century & the rise of medical technology, to today's landmark cases of people's right to this has important information when your own loved-one says: "Enough!"

Medicine Cards: The Discovery of Power through the Ways of Animals
   by Jamie Sams and David Carson.
   Illustrated by Angela C. Werneke.
   Publisher: Bear & Company 1988   ISBN: 093968053X
   Subjects: 1) Indians of North America.
             2) Healing with Animal Powers.
             3) Fortune-telling cards.

The exquisite illustrations in both this deck of cards & book re-create a whimsical & instructive way of learning through North American First People's myths. Each day's layout offers a way through the thick veils of modern daily life into the fresh air of a wider, wilder world.

Perfect Endings: a conscious approach to dying & death by Robert Sachs
   Publisher: Healing Arts Press 1998   ISBN: 0892817798
   Subjects: 1) Death–Psychological aspects.
             2) Terminally ill–Psychology
             3) Case studies–Family relationships

This one shows us how death can expand our experience of living. All the strength & wisdom of our lifetime are called forth as we move thru our dying. Really helpful in maintaining a broader view of it all & listening to our beloved Poppa. Reviewed on rebeccasreads.com.

Questions & Answers on Death & Dying
by Elisabeth Kübler-Ross.
Publisher: Macmillan 1974   ISBN: 0020891504
Subjects: 1) Terminal care.
2) Death.
3) Understanding the dying patient.

40 years ago this author shocked us by writing & teaching about the gentle art of dying. A compilation of the most frequently asked questions(FAQs) this revered author & teacher faces at every one of her classes & seminars. The questions are as daffy & serious as any we had.

Spirit-Walking
by Carolyn Stearns
Publisher: IM Press 1996   ISBN: 0965465136
Subjects: 1) Voices from Beyond Death.
2) Emotional comfort.
3) Visions, Poetry.

Stories & poems relating to & recounted by recently deceased loved-ones, people & pets. A compassionate guide to bereavement, teaching us how to overcome our fears about death & loss. Reviewed on rebeccasreads.com.

The New Chain-Reference Bible: King James Version
Edited by Frank Charles Thompson
Publisher: B. B. Kirkbridge Bible Co. 1934   No ISBN
Subjects: 1) Spirituality
         2) Psychology
         3) Reading Primer

Poppa's edition was marked throughout, especially The Psalms. It was his book of choice since he was called to the words of his Savior.

The Power of Myth
by Joseph Campbell and Bill Moyers.
Betty Sue Flowers, Editor
Publisher: Doubleday 1988   ISBN: 0385247737
Subjects: 1) Myths and their meaning.
         2) History of religion and rites.
         3) Thoughts about consciousness.

These conversations between two thoughtful men are about how our global mythologies have meaning as we face life & struggle, consciousness & death. In his questions, Bill spoke for me; in his answers, Joseph lit my Path.

The Third Eye
by T. Lobsang Rampa
Publisher: Ballantine Books 1995 ISBN: 0345340388
Subjects: 1) Tibetan Buddhism
2) Spiritual training
3) Reincarnation

A wonder-filled fact-cum-fiction memoir of a young Tibetan monk's life. I learnt to see auras & how to crack open the iron egg in which my mind & soul resided. It is where I first read about seeing the Light of the Spirit & from that I was able to do so at Poppa's passing.

When the Drummers Were Women: A Spiritual History of Rhythm
by Layne Redmond
Publisher: Three Rivers Press 1997 ISBN: 0609801287
Subjects: 1) Pre-Christian religious practices.
2) Women's religious rites.
3) Women and the power of the drums.

A scholarly & inspiring exploration & memoir into the power of the Call of the Drum, from the earliest archeological finds to modern practices. A gift from my son with whom, on occasion, I still drum. As a woman who answered the Call of the Drum, this book made a difference in my spiritual & ceremonial life. Reviewed on rebeccasreads.com.

For Children

Someone I Love Died
by Christine Harder Tangvald
Illustrated by Benton Mahan
Publisher: David C. Cook Pub. 1988 ISBN: 1555134904
Subjects: 1) Death–Juvenile literature.
               2) Christianity–Juvenile.
               3) Death–Religious aspects.

This is a charming little book in the Please Help Me, God series. Things to think about, & how to recognize grief.

The Goodbye Boat
by Mary Joslin. Illustrator Claire St. Louis Little
Publisher: Eerdmans Books 1998 ISBN: 080285186X
Subjects: 1) Children and Death–Juvenile literature
               2) Saying goodbye
               3) Death

Saying goodbye to someone you love is always hard. Saying goodbye when someone you love dies is perhaps the hardest thing of all. Beautiful pictures with a lot to think about. Reviewed on rebeccasreads.com.

* * * * *

While all these books, in one way of another, smoothed the wrinkles from our worried brows, none of them really addressed the hands-on, intimate details of taking care of an elder as do books about baby care. Perhaps, by the time we've reached the age when it is our turn to take care of our parents, as they cared for us in our childhood, we're expected to already know how to tend an adult human?

While cruising the Web, I came upon some truly informative & supportive sites. Keywords: death and dying at home.

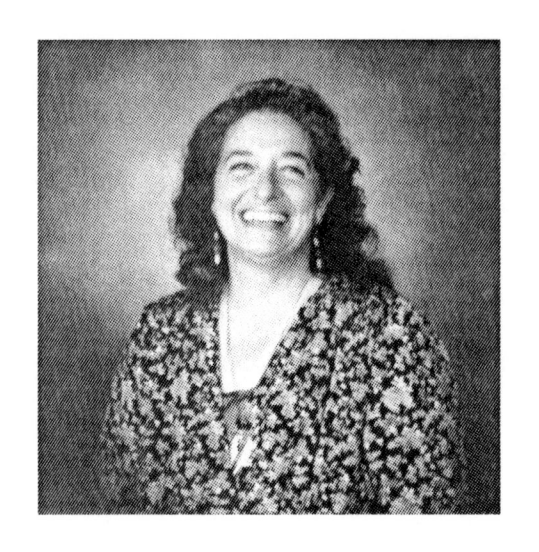

About the Author

Rebecca Brown, an adopted war orphan, was raised in England. At age 22, she emigrated to Chicago, Illinois, where she worked with Rabbi Marx and Dr. King, in the Civil Rights Movement. Later she joined the Counter Culture. When she moved to the Northwest, to give her children a small town schooling, she became the Managing Editor of the *Townsend Letter for Doctors*.

Most recently, Rebecca and her husband, David, created **rebeccasreads.com**, an award-winning website devoted to the love of reading and writing.

0-595-22750-3

Printed in the United States
6775